Angel Shannon's

STICK OF BUTTER COOKBOOK

· · · · · · · · · · · · · · · · · ·

CFI
Springville, Utah

ISBN 13: 978-1-59955-009-1

Published by CFI, an imprint of Cedar Fort, Inc., 2373 W. 700 S., Springville, UT, 84663
Distributed by Cedar Fort, Inc. www.cedarfort.com

LIBRARY OF CONGRESS CATALOGING-IN-PUBLICATION DATA

Shannon, Angel, 1959-
    Stick of Butter Cookbook / Angel Shannon.
        p. cm.
    ISBN-13: 978-1-59955-009-1
    1. Cookery (Butter) I. Title.

    TX759.5.B87S53 2007
    641.3'72--dc22

                                      2006039288

Cover design by Nicole Williams
Edited and typeset by Annaliese B. Cox
Cover design © 2007 by Lyle Mortimer

Printed in China

10 9 8 7 6 5 4 3 2 1

Printed on acid-free paper

Dedication

This cookbook is proudly dedicated to Dana Robinson for his undying support, love, and vision. Also to Cedar Fort's Lee Nelson for his patience and for allowing me the luxury of following my dreams.

But most of all, to my fellow home chefs who never forget that cooking is like "therapy in a skillet." May each recipe you follow lead to happiness and love around your own kitchen table!

Table of Contents

Acknowledgments

To my sister Julie and my best friends Diana and Marci, now known as "The Butter Babes" after spending hours helping me double check these recipes so that none of us will be sorry!

To my husband Bill, for his love—of me and of butter—and for always being willing to try "just one more bite." To George Severson of ABC4's Good Things Utah, my friend and mentor who taught me to believe in myself and not to let the bumps in life pull me off course. To my cat Scooter, who fancies himself a dairy connoisseur.

And, finally, to the 128 sticks of butter that were sacrificed in the making of this cookbook. I loved you all in so many different ways.

Long Live Butter!

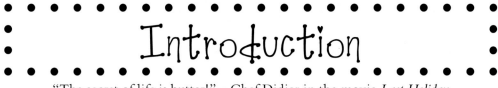

Introduction

"The secret of life is butter!"—Chef Didier in the movie *Last Holiday*

There's nothing quite as pleasing as a slice of freshly baked bread slathered with honey butter or as satisfying as rich butter cookies dunked in ice-cold milk. If it's so good, then why do we feel so bad for loving that golden ray of sunshine melted over the top of a fluffy baked potato?

I'll tell you why. Because the margarine marketing machine is hard at work convincing us that butter is bad for you. The United States Department of Agriculture says it's bad for you. Your health-conscious neighbor says it's bad for you. For crying out loud, hasn't anybody ever heard of portion control? Butter contains no trans fatty acids, and it's rich in vitamins A, D, and E. It's also chock-full of CLA, which recent studies show helps to normalize fat accumulation in the human body.

The trouble with butter is simple. It's so delicious that we have eight cookies instead of two. We put two tablespoons of butter on top of our fresh green beans instead of just one. Let's make a deal. I'll share all of these butter recipes with you if you'll promise to eat just one croissant, have only one bowl of butter-topped clam chowder, and when it comes to those Sunday pancakes—you might want to just use the butter-flavored syrup instead of half the stick!

Well . . . you can try at least. Enjoy!

—*Angel Shannon*

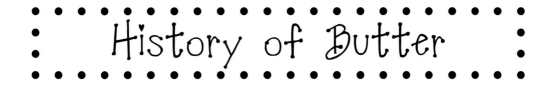

History of Butter

The background of butter is as much a mystery as it is a history. The stories weave their way though Asia, India, and Scandinavia and onward into Germany and Switzerland. Was it the ancient Hebrews or the dwellers of Asiatic India who first discovered butter? Some say it was wandering nomads, while others insist it was Syrians who churned the first batch.

Made from the milk of cows, goats, buffaloes, yaks, and horses, its many uses range from lamp oil to medicine and even as an ingredient in cosmetics. Did you know it has even been used to coat skin for protection against wind and bugs? And some cultures have used butter for sacrificial worship rituals. Butter's allure was so valued in ancient times that it was often used as currency or traded for other items at the local street market. Ancient Greeks used olive oil to cook with and used butter as an ointment!

In Tibet, Buddhist monks create intricate and colorful yak butter sculptures as part of their path to enlightenment. In Russia, the annual Butter Week says good-bye to winter and welcomes the warmer spring days by offering visitors pancakes with honey, fresh cream, caviar, and butter. It's a culinary treasure as old as King Tut's Tomb.

In 1493, Christopher Columbus brought cows from Europe to the Western hemisphere. By the 1500s, stray cows from ranches in Mexico had migrated north into what is now the United States, and with them came sweet cream and plenty of milk. Colonial and early American fare included rich wedding cakes, doughnuts, and baked apple crunch filled with butter made fresh on the family farm.

By the 1860s, Thomas Jefferson's daily breakfast always included butter slathered over Monticello Muffins, and his dinner most definitely included cream sauces of some sort—whether over roast lamb or as a dessert pudding. During his years as minister to France, he made sure his slaves were schooled in the art of French cooking, which, of course, is all about butter, cream, and sauces.

History of Butter

Over the centuries, people have preserved butter by wrapping it in leaves and then covering the leaves with cow dung to dry. It's been hidden from invaders, and ripened and stored in Irish peat bogs. Butter has been transported in the back of wagons with freshly cut grass layered over the top. Butter has been canned, wrapped in cheesecloth, and, finally, in the late 1800s, somebody came up with the brilliant idea of using paraffin paper—and the timing couldn't have been better. By 1894 the "World's Largest Creamery" in Vermont was making 25,000 lbs. of butter daily.

Churning butter started out with heavy cream in a container attached to a saddle bag on the back of a spirited horse for a few miles. Or was it a goatskin filled with cream and agitated by primitive rocker churns? Churns have been made from glass, stoneware, tin, and wood. The dash churn is the one we usually imagine pioneer women using in the Old West. Modern industrial churns can produce one ton of butter per hour.

The first exhibition style butter sculpture in America was carved by Mrs. Carolyn Brooks for our Centennial Exhibition in 1876. Ten years later, the definition and standards for butter in the United States was set by Congress; it was the only food with that distinction prior to the enactment of the Food, Drug, and Cosmetic Act of 1938.

Now, in the twenty-first century, butter has been a kitchen staple right alongside flour and milk. Did you spread butter on your toast or banana bread this morning? Did your Mom spread butter on your sandwich bread or pour it all over your Jiffy-Pop? Were you piling butter on your baked potato along with sour cream, chives, and cheese at dinner? If so, you're a proud member of the Butter Generation! On average, each American consumes about 4 lbs. of butter a year—so you're in good company. It must have something to do with the old Norwegian proverb: "Cookies are made of butter and love."

Nutrition

It was once thought that it was healthier to use margarine than butter, but recent studies indicate that margarine users, feeling safer, tend to use margarine more liberally and thus ingest more fat (Revised from Rubin, *The Kitchen Answer Book*).

• • •

Myth: Saturated fat clogs arteries

Truth: The fatty acids found in artery clogs are mostly unsaturated (74%) of which 41% are polyunsaturated (*Lancet* 1994 344:1195).

• • •

Cholesterol is especially important to our brains. That's right, today's "most hated" substance is essential to human brain function. In fact, infants need a constant supply of cholesterol during brain development which is why mother's breast milk is so high in it. Modern science tripped over itself somehow when it named cholesterol the bugaboo of heart disease. Nature doesn't make that kind of mistake—but man does (Valentine, *Facts on Fats and Oils*).

• • •

A series of feeding experiments on rats showed differences in their nutritive value of common fats. The rats which received butterfat grew better than the rats fed vegetable oils, were better in appearance, and had better reproductive capacity. . . . these findings are significant to the knowledge of nutrition because they indicate additional reasons why milk fat has superior value for human diets (Price, *Nutrition and Physical Degeneration*).

• • •

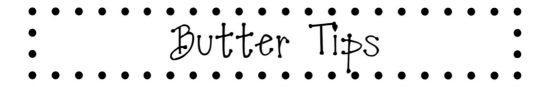

Butter Tips

Baking

- If you're making cake batter or cookie dough, start by creaming the room temperature butter with the sugar.

- For pastry dough, such as pie or tart shell dough, butter should be cold before cutting into dry ingredients.

- Butter picks up the flavor of anything around it or mixed into it—a characteristic that can be a nuisance in the refrigerator! However, butter's ability to morph into a sweet and creamy cinnamon-sugar spread or into a garlicky, flavorful herb spread gives us even more reason to love it.

Making Butter

Homemade Butter:

- Makin' butter with the kids . . . you don't need an old-fashioned churn, just do a little salsa dancin'! Pour at least a pint of heavy cream into a plastic jar and make sure the lid's on really tight. Everybody gets a turn shaking up the cream. They can dance and jump, and in just twenty minutes or so, you can strain off the liquid, add a pinch of salt, and chill your very own homemade butter.

Whipped Butter:

- Put 1 stick softened butter into a bowl; beat with electric mixer until it's fluffy. Flavor with garlic oil, chopped roasted peppers, pesto, etc. Cover and store in fridge.

Butter Tips

Clarified butter:

- Cut butter in small chunks so it will melt at a lower temperature.
- Melt slowly in saucepan until the solids separate from the fat. By solids, I mean the milk proteins and salt (it also eliminates the water). Most of the solids will drop to the bottom, but a white foam layer will form on top.
- Do not stir. Carefully remove saucepan from the burner and spoon the foam off the top.
- Put in an oven-safe glass container in the oven at its lowest setting. Glass is better because it allows you to monitor the process. Do not stir!
- Cool in the fridge for at least an hour and do not disturb the bowl until the middle fat layer has solidified.
- Lift out the solidified fat disk. Scrape off as much of foam and slimy bottom layer as possible without damaging the disk. Finish the cleaning step by quickly rinsing the disk under cold, running tap water. Pat dry with a paper towel.
- Clarified butter keeps longer because the milk solids aren't there to sour! It can be used for sautéing, tossing with steamed vegetables, or for brushing on poached fish. One pound of butter equals about 1½ cups clarified butter. (Revised from Rubin, *The Kitchen Answer Book*)

To make your own spreadable creation, add the one of the following per stick of butter:

- 3 Tbsp. orange marmalade
- ½ cup crushed nuts (like macadamia or almonds) + 1 teaspoon of honey
- 1 large roast garlic clove, minced
- 1½ teaspoon of assorted fresh savory herbs like basil, rosemary, thyme, or oregano

Storage

- Butter tends to pick up odors from foods stored around it in the refrigerator. Make sure it's covered tightly, and it's best to keep butter in its original storage carton.

- Butter can be refrigerated for up to 4 months.

- Butter can be frozen for up to 1 year. Make sure you use thawed butter immediately.

Butter Tips

Butter Grades

U.S. Grade AA Butter:

- Delicate, sweet flavor, with a fine, highly pleasing aroma
- Made from high-quality, fresh sweet cream
- Smooth, creamy texture with good spreadability
- Salt completely dissolved and blended

U.S. Grade A Butter:

- Pleasing flavor
- Made from fresh sweet cream
- Fairly smooth texture
- Rates close to the top grade

U.S. Grade B Butter:

- May have slightly acid flavor
- Generally made from selected sour cream
- Acceptable by many consumers

Source: WebExhibits.org

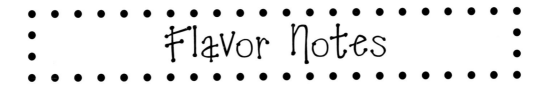

Flavor Notes

Over 120 different compounds contribute to butter's flavor, but only two classes of compounds are responsible for the most characteristic flavor notes: methyl ketones and lactones. Both compounds are present in butter at levels below detection, or below their Flavor Threshold Value (FTV).

When butter is heated, however, concentrations of both compounds rise above their FTV and the two compounds react synergistically, providing the rich, cooked butter flavor commonly associated with numerous entrées.

Butter works synergistically with other flavors and can provide a primary flavor in fish or poultry entrées. In fact, butter sauces have become a standard for fish entrées. Butter can also provide rich background flavor notes in entrée stuffings and sauces. Chicken Kiev is a classic example of this application.

Butter can be heated to different temperatures to provide cooked and smoked flavors that are often absent in microwavable foods. Slightly overheated butter ("brown" melt) creates roasted, cooked flavors which complement entrées of roasted meat or poultry and gravies. Butter that is overheated to the "dark brown" melt stage contributes smoked flavor notes which complement smoked fish and turkey entrées, as well as barbecue-style meals.

Source: wisdairy.com

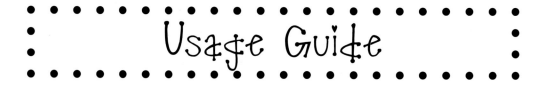

Usage Guide

All flour is all-purpose unless otherwise noted.

All butter is unsalted unless otherwise noted.

Pay attention to commas, please!

    1 cup flour, sifted = measure then sift
    1 cup sifted flour = sift then measure
    Tbsp.—tablespoon
    tsp.—teaspoon

All ingredients are listed in the same order that they are used in each recipe's directions.

Pasta *al dente* is cooked just enough to retain a somewhat firm texture.

Measurement Equivalents

    1 tablespoon (Tbsp.) = 3 teaspoons (tsp.)
    ¼ cup = 4 tablespoons
    1 cup = 48 teaspoons
    1 cup = 16 tablespoons
    8 fluid ounces (fl. oz.) = 1 cup
    1 pint (pt.) = 2 cups
    1 quart (qt.) = 2 pints
    4 cups = 1 quart
    1 gallon (gal.) = 4 quarts
    16 ounces (oz.) = 1 pound (lb.)

Appetizers

Creamy Pesto Dip
Date & Walnut Roll-ups
French Bread Fantastic
Encore Italian Barbecued Shrimp
Mushroom & Artichoke Garlic Cream
Spinach Snacks
Olive Party Bites

"As for butter versus margarine, I trust cows more than chemists"

—Nutritionist Joan Gussow

Creamy Pesto Dip

2 sticks butter, softened
1 (8 oz.) pkg. cream cheese, room temperature
1 (8–10 oz.) jar pesto

Whip butter and cream cheese together.

Line a 10-inch deep dish pie pan with plastic wrap, leaving plenty hanging over edge. Spread half of cream cheese mixture into bottom of pan, then spread the entire jar of pesto over all. Top with the remaining half of cream cheese mixture. Wrap tightly in plastic wrap, pulling sides up over the top. Cover and chill overnight in refrigerator.

To serve, carefully pull plastic wrap away from top, invert mix onto serving dish, and pull the rest of the wrap off. Serve with butter crackers (like Ritz crackers) or as a topping for baked potatoes.

Date & Walnut Roll-ups

I've been known to add red or green food coloring to the dough for a little extra holiday touch.

    2 sticks butter
    1 (8 oz.) pkg. cream cheese
    2 cups flour
    ¼ tsp. salt
      cornstarch
      powdered sugar
      pitted dates (35–40, whole)
      walnut halves

Cream butter and cream cheese together; blend in flour and salt. Chill dough for at least 2 hours.

Roll chilled dough into rectangle ⅛ inch thick using cornstarch to keep dough from sticking to surface. Sprinkle with powdered sugar and cut into 1×3 inch strips.

Push walnut half into each pitted date; place one stuffed date on center of each strip; roll up. Position "seam side" down on a cookie sheet. Bake at 375 degrees for 15–20 minutes. Dust with powdered sugar while still warm.

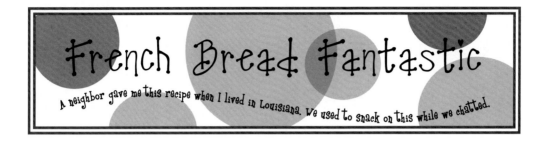

French Bread Fantastic

A neighbor gave me this recipe when I lived in Louisiana. We used to snack on this while we chatted.

1 large loaf French bread
1 stick butter, softened
½ cup mayonnaise
2 cups shredded sharp cheddar cheese
½ cup chopped green onions
½ cup chopped black olives
¼ tsp. garlic powder

Slice French bread in half horizontally and scoop out just a little bit of the bread from each half. Place loaf on foil lined cookie sheet. Preheat oven to 350 degrees.

Mix butter and mayo together until smooth. Mix in cheese, onions, olives, and garlic powder. Spread mixture on both cut sides. Bake for 15–20 minutes or until lightly toasted and spread is bubbly.

This recipe freezes well. Just wrap in foil before baking and stick it in the freezer for up to 4 months. To bake, just thaw on countertop and follow above directions.

Encore Italian Barbecued Shrimp

...The perfect finish for a night out on the town...

4 lbs. medium to large shrimp in the shell, without heads
2 sticks butter, sliced up
1 whole head of garlic, peeled and chopped
1 oz. pepper
2 Tbsp. Tabasco
1 Tbsp. paprika
1 Tbsp. dried oregano
1 Tbsp. dried rosemary

Rinse shrimp in cold water; drain well and pat dry with paper towels. Place them in a large, deep baking dish. Sprinkle butter slices, chopped garlic, pepper, Tabasco, paprika, oregano, and rosemary over top of shrimp. Bake at 375 degrees about 15–20 minutes (shells will be pink).

Serve with crusty bread and your favorite beverage.

Mushroom & Artichoke Garlic Cream

8 large mushrooms, sliced
2 cloves garlic, crushed
1 stick butter
4 Tbsp. flour
1 cup half and half
1 tsp. dry mustard
1½ cups artichoke hearts, chopped (canned or frozen—heated up in own juices)
½ cup shredded Parmesan cheese
Butter crackers (like Ritz crackers) for serving
1 Tbsp. chopped chives

Melt butter in large saucepan; sauté mushrooms and garlic until tender. Remove from heat. Add flour and cook until bubbly; then add half and half and mustard. Simmer and stir until thick. Add sautéed mushrooms, garlic, and warmed chopped artichoke hearts. Sprinkle with Parmesan cheese. Serve on crackers with chives sprinkled on top.

Tip: You can use toast points or mini pastry shells in place of crackers if desired.

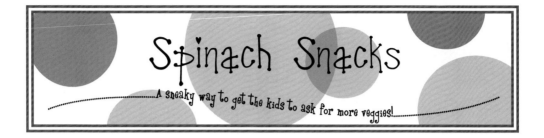

Spinach Snacks

A sneaky way to get the kids to ask for more veggies!

    2 (10 oz.) pkgs. frozen spinach, drained well
    2 cups seasoned croutons
    ½ cup Parmesan cheese
    1½ sticks butter, melted
    ½ cup chopped onion
    ½ tsp. salt
    ½ pepper
    ½ garlic powder
    ½ thyme

Combine all ingredients; roll into 1 inch balls. Bake 15–20 minutes at 350 degrees until lightly browned.

Olive Party Bites

...Fun little pop-in-your-mouth appetizers. Everyone will rave!...

    1 stick butter, softened
    ½ lb. room temperature American cheese, cut into small pieces or shredded
    1 cup flour
    ½ tsp. salt
    ⅛ tsp. pepper
    1 tsp. onion powder
    1 tsp. paprika
    2 Tbsp. dried parsley
    36 small stuffed olives, drained well

Cream butter and cheese together. Blend in flour, salt, pepper, onion powder, paprika, and parsley. Shape 1 tsp. of pastry mix around each olive, covering completely. Roll between palms into a ball. Arrange balls on shallow pan (close but not touching) and freeze. At serving time, bake at 400 degrees until golden (about 15 minutes). Serve hot.

Breads

Angel food Pound Cake
Apple Spice Bread
Cheddar Cracker-Biscuits
Garlic Loaves
Gooey-nutty Pull-aparts
Hawaiian Nut Bread
Holiday Gift Bread
Jolly Jelly-filled Biscuits

Keep Eatin' Corn Bread
Lemon Parsley Sourdough Rolls
Lunch Stop Pear Muffins
Maple Walnut Muffins
Onion Bread
Orange Marmalade Bread
Parmesan Bread
Sweet Potato Rolls

Keep your words as soft and sweet as butter...............

because it's just possible you may have to eat them later on.

Angel Food Pound Cake

Is it a cake or is it bread?
Slather it with honey butter or cut into cubes and serve sprinkled with fresh berries and cream.

  1 stick butter
  ¼ cup sugar
  2 cups cake flour
  2 tsp. baking powder
  1 cup milk
  1 egg, beaten

Cream butter and sugar. Sift together flour and baking powder. Alternately add creamed mixture with the milk; blend in egg. Bake in lightly greased 9×5 loaf pan for 30 minutes. Serve piping hot for best flavor. Reheats easily in microwave or oven.

(I've always wanted to try this, cubed, in a bread pudding style dessert. If you get time, try it and let me know if it's good!)

Apple Spice Bread

Makes a terrific gift if you can stop eating it yourself!

1 stick butter, softened
1 cup sugar
2 eggs
2 cups peeled, cored, and finely chopped apples
1 tsp. cinnamon
1 tsp. salt
1 tsp. vanilla
1 Tbsp. lemon zest
⅔ cup chopped walnuts or pecans
2 cups flour
1 tsp. baking soda
½ tsp. cloves

Cream butter and sugar together; add eggs one at a time until well mixed.

Mix in apples by hand; then stir in cinnamon, salt, vanilla, lemon zest, and nuts.

Sift together flour, baking soda and cloves. Mix a little at a time into apple batter until well blended.

Pour into a lightly greased and floured 9×5×3 loaf pan. Bake at 350 degrees for 50 minutes. Cool in pan for 15 minutes and turn out onto rack.

Cheddar Cracker-Biscuits

These will remind you of Cheese Nips. Heavenly served with a green salad or floating on top of tomato soup.

　1 cup flour
　⅓ cup buttermilk
　½ tsp. baking powder
　1 cup shredded sharp cheddar cheese
　1 stick butter
　　dash of cayenne
　　garlic salt to taste

Mix all ingredients in a bowl, working into dough. Roll out on floured board to about ¼ inch thick; cut with 2 inch round cutter and place on lightly greased and floured cookie sheet. Bake in a 425 degree oven for 10–13 minutes or until light golden brown.

Tip: Try pushing a few pine nuts into the top of each round before baking.

Garlic Loaves

½ cup olive oil
2 sticks butter
8 cloves garlic, crushed
1 tsp. crushed oregano
1 tsp. crushed basil
¼ tsp. crushed dried red chilies
2 loaves French bread, sliced horizontally and toasted

Combine olive oil and butter in skillet. Heat over medium until hot. Sauté garlic until gold; reduce heat and add oregano, basil, and chilies. Simmer 15 minutes. Pour mixture equally into two 9×13 baking dishes. Place 2 bread halves, cut side down, into each dish. Let stand a few minutes to soak up garlic butter. Turn cut side up and toast at 400 degrees for 7–10 minutes or until crispy and golden.

Before serving, cut into 2 inch slices.

Gooey-nutty Pull-aparts

Experiment by sprinkling coconut, raisins, dates, or craisins into the topping. Hop in everybody!

Dough

- 2 pkgs. dry yeast
- ½ cup warm water (100–110 degrees)
- ¾ cup milk
- ½ stick butter
- 1 tsp. salt
- 1 egg, lightly beaten
- ¼ cup sugar
- 3¼ cups flour

Topping

- 1½ sticks butter
- 1 cup brown sugar
- ¾ cup chopped pecans
- 1 Tbsp. dark corn syrup
- 1 Tbsp. water

Stir yeast and warm water together in large mixing bowl and set side. Heat milk, butter, and salt in saucepan until just warm, stirring constantly. Slowly pour into yeast water, mixing well as you go. Add egg, sugar, and flour. Scrape down sides of bowl. Cover with kitchen towel and let rise in a warm place for 30 minutes.

While dough is rising, prepare the topping. In medium saucepan, blend all topping ingredients together over low heat just until butter melts. Grease sides of 9×13×2 pan and pour butter mixture into the bottom. Stir down batter after 30 minutes and drop by tablespoon over topping. Cover and let rise 30 more minutes. Bake at 375 degrees for 20–25 minutes or until golden brown.

Loosen sides with knife and cool for 10 minutes. Re-check sides to be sure the bread is not stuck before inverting onto wax paper.

Hawaiian Nut Bread

2 (20 oz.) cans crushed pineapple
2 cups bran flakes cereal
1 cup sour cream
¾ cup honey, divided
2 eggs
1 Tbsp. cinnamon

½ tsp. nutmeg
1 stick butter, melted
3⅓ cups biscuit mix (like Bisquick)
1 cup chopped macadamia nuts or walnuts (reserve ¼ cup)

Drain pineapple, reserving ½ cup of the juice.

In a large bowl combine pineapple, reserved juice, bran flakes, and sour cream. Let stand 15 minutes or until bran flakes are softened.

Stir in ½ cup honey, eggs, cinnamon, and nutmeg. Mix well. Blend in melted butter. Add biscuit mix and mix ingredients together. Stir in nuts. Spoon into 2 well-greased 9×9×2 pans. Top with reserved nuts and drizzle with a little extra honey (about ¼ cup, more if desired). Bake at 375 degrees for 35–40 minutes or until toothpick inserted in center comes out clean.

Cool and top with whipped cream or ice cream if desired.

To make muffins: Follow recipe as above except use a regular muffin tin. Use muffin papers and fill cups ⅔ full. Top with nuts and honey as above. Cook at 375 degrees for 20–25 minutes or until a toothpick inserted into one of the muffins comes out clean.

Yield: Two 9×9 loaves or 25–30 regular sized muffins. This recipe may be easily cut in half.

Holiday Gift Bread

1 stick butter, softened
1 cup sugar
2 eggs
1½ tsp. vanilla
2 cups flour
1 tsp. baking soda
½ tsp. salt
1 cup mashed bananas
1 can (11 oz.) mandarin oranges, drained

¾ cup coconut
¾ cup chocolate chips
½ cup chopped or slivered nuts
   (almonds, walnuts, pecans, etc.)
¼ cup chopped red maraschino
   cherries
¼ cup chopped green maraschino
   cherries
½ cup chopped dates

Cream butter and sugar in large bowl; add eggs and vanilla, mixing well. Sift flour, baking soda, and salt onto a sheet of wax paper. Add flour mix to creamed mixture, alternating with bananas; mix in oranges, coconut, chocolate chips, ¼ cup nuts, cherries, and dates. Pour into two greased 8×4×2 inch loaf pans and sprinkle remaining nuts on top. Bake at 350 degrees for 50 minutes or until toothpick comes out clean. Cool 10 minutes before removing from pans.

Tip: You can substitute raisins or dried cranberries for dates if preferred.

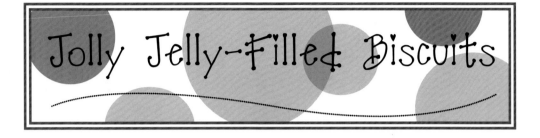

Jolly Jelly-Filled Biscuits

    1 (12 oz.) can refrigerated biscuits
 ¾ cup sugar
    1 Tbsp. cinnamon
 ½ tsp. nutmeg
    1 stick butter, melted
 ⅓ cup raspberry jelly (or preferred flavor)

Prepare and bake biscuits according to directions.

Mix sugar and spices in small bowl. Pour melted butter into a second bowl.

Place a piece of parchment or wax paper on countertop and as soon as biscuits come out of the oven, dip in butter, roll well in sugar mixture, and place on paper.

Stick small paring knife into the side of biscuit until it slides most of the way through.

To fill, put jelly in either a baster or a pastry bag with a small tip and carefully insert into the side of each biscuit, squeezing small amount of jelly inside. Refill as needed. If you're filling while hot, tilt the biscuit slightly so that jelly doesn't run back out.

These are excellent warm or cold.

Keep Eatin' Corn Bread

You can only guess how this rich and cheesy recipe got its name!

1 cup sugar
2 sticks butter
4 eggs
1 can cream style corn
1 can green chilies (not hot!) with juice
1 cup shredded Monterey Jack cheese
1 cup cheddar cheese
1 cup flour
4 tsp. baking powder
½ tsp. salt
1 cup yellow cornmeal

Mix sugar, butter, and eggs together; add corn, chilies (with juice), and cheeses and mix well. Add flour, baking powder, salt, and cornmeal. Bake in a lightly sprayed 9×9 cake pan. Bake at 375 degrees for about 30–35 minutes.

Tip: Place parchment paper in bottom of pan just to be sure the cornbread releases easily.

Lemon Parsley Sourdough Rolls

A nice touch for a summer salad meal

8 large French sourdough rolls
1 stick butter, softened
2 Tbsp. finely chopped fresh parsley
1 Tbsp. freshly squeezed lemon juice
1½ tsp. grated lemon rind
    sweet paprika

Preheat oven to 350 degrees. Mix butter, parsley, juice, and rind. Cut rolls in half horizontally and spread with mixture. Sprinkle with paprika. Wrap in aluminum foil and heat in oven for 15 minutes.

Tip: I like to sprinkle prepared salad seasoning over my rolls, like Salad Supreme or Emeril's Bam It! Salad Seasoning. If you want, sprinkle with Parmesan cheese and grill to a golden brown cut side down, instead of baking.

Lunch Stop Pear Muffins

Makes 24 muffins—so you can eat some, freeze some, and give some to neighbors...

Muffins
- 3 cups flour
- 1½ tsp. baking powder
- ½ tsp. baking soda
- ¾ tsp. salt
- 1 stick butter
- 1½ cups sugar
- 2 eggs
- ½ cup fresh orange juice
- 1½ cups chopped pears
- 2 Tbsp. grated orange rind
- 1½ cups bran flakes
- ⅓–½ cup chopped walnuts

Topping
- 3 Tbsp. butter
- ½ cup plus 1 Tbsp. brown sugar
- 1 tsp. mace
- 3 Tbsp. flour

Sift together flour, baking powder, baking soda, and salt. Set aside.

Cream butter; add sugar and beat until fluffy. Add eggs one at a time, beating well after each. Add dry ingredients alternately with orange juice, pears, and orange rind; mix well. Fold in bran flakes and chopped nuts.

Lightly grease and flour 2 muffin tins (12 ea.). Preheat oven to 350 degrees. Fill each muffin cup half full of batter.

Make topping by cutting butter into brown sugar, mace, and flour.

Sprinkle topping on each muffin and bake at 350 degrees for 10–13 minutes or until toothpick comes out mostly clean. Cool in pans for 10 minutes. Turn out onto racks to finish cooling.

Tip: To freeze, wrap muffins in plastic wrap and place in freezer bag.

Maple Walnut Muffins

2¼ cups flour
1 tsp. baking powder
½ tsp. baking soda
½ tsp. salt
1 stick butter
2 Tbsp. maple syrup
1 tsp. maple flavoring
2 eggs, lightly beaten
1 (8 oz.) carton plain yogurt
1 cup sugar
¼ cup chopped walnuts

Preheat oven to 350 degrees.

In large bowl, mix together flour, baking powder, baking soda, and salt; cut in butter until mixture resembles cornmeal.

Whisk together maple syrup, flavoring, eggs, yogurt, and sugar. Mix in dry ingredients, stirring until just blended. Lightly mix in chopped nuts.

Spoon batter evenly into 18 greased muffin cups (use paper cup liners if desired). Bake 20–25 minutes.

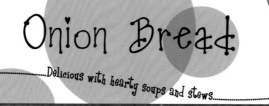

Onion Bread

Delicious with hearty soups and stews

2 cups flour
3 Tbsp. baking powder
½ tsp. salt
1 stick butter
1 egg
   onion slices (¼ inch thick)
¼ tsp. salt
⅓ cup mayonnaise
   celery seeds

Combine flour, baking powder, salt and butter blending well. Put egg in measuring cup and fill to ⅔ cup with water; whisk. Slowly beat into first mixture, blending well. Pour dough into greased glass dish (8 inch round × 2 inch deep). Press well to edges with slightly hollowed center. Cover with onion slices, overlapping edges. Sprinkle with salt and smooth mayonnaise evenly over top. Sprinkle with celery seeds and bake at 350 degrees for 30 minutes or until golden brown.

Orange Marmalade Bread

    1 stick butter, softened
    ½ cup brown sugar
    2 eggs
    1 (10 oz.) jar orange marmalade
 2¾ cups flour
    2 tsp. baking powder
    1 tsp. salt
    ½ tsp. baking soda
    ½ cup orange juice, unsweetened
    ½ cup walnuts, chopped

Cream margarine and sugar until light and fluffy. Add eggs one at a time and mix well. Blend in marmalade. Combine flour, baking powder, salt, and baking soda. Add dry mixture to creamed margarine mix alternately with orange juice. Stir in nuts. Pour into greased and floured loaf pan. Bake at 350 degrees for about 1 hour. Test with toothpick for doneness. Cool 15 minutes before removing from pan.

Parmesan Bread

This is a hearty no-nonsense pull-apart bread. Think about adding a layer of crispy fried bacon bits—delish!

1 cup shredded Parmesan cheese	3 Tbsp. wheat germ
2 Tbsp. parsley flakes	¼ cup sour cream
2 tsp. dried chives	1 egg
¼ tsp. paprika	¼ cup milk
3 cups biscuit mix (like Bisquick)	1 stick butter, melted

Loosely blend Parmesan cheese, parsley, chives, and paprika together and set aside.

In a large bowl, mix together biscuit mix and wheat germ. Whisk sour cream, egg, and milk in a separate bowl; add back into the biscuit mixture, blending well until a stiff dough ball can be formed. Knead about 10 times; shape into 1-inch balls.

Dip dough balls into melted butter then roll in the Parmesan blend. Drop evenly into a greased tube pan, sprinkling a little cheese coating between layers. Sprinkle any leftover Parmesan mixture over the top.

Bake at 400 degrees for 15–20 minutes or until golden brown. Cool; loosen from sides of pan and invert onto serving plate.

Tip: Put a small bowl of warmed marinara sauce in the center of this bread round. Makes for a pretty presentation!

Sweet Potato Rolls

¾ cups mashed sweet potatoes
1 stick butter, melted
½ cup milk
1½ cup flour
1 tsp. pumpkin pie spice
1 Tbsp. baking powder
½ tsp. salt

Preheat oven to 450 degrees

Combine first 3 ingredients in large bowl. Sift flour, pumpkin pie spice, baking powder, and salt together and add to sweet potato mixture, blending well.

Roll dough ½ inch thick on floured surface; cut with 2-inch biscuit cutter. Place on lightly greased baking sheet. Sprinkle with cinnamon and sugar if desired.

Bake on top rack 12–15 minutes or until brown. Delicious with Pecan Honey Butter!

Breakfast

Sunshine Almond Scones
Danish Breakfast Pastry
Holiday Sausage Bake
Huevos Ole
Lazy Morning French Toast
Laid-back Butterhorns
Sausage & Cheese Strudel

Old recipes can refer to "butter the size of a walnut."

In today's terms, that means 2 tablespoons................

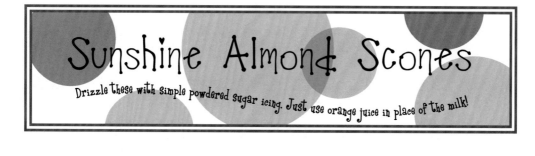

Sunshine Almond Scones

Drizzle these with simple powdered sugar icing. Just use orange juice in place of the milk!

½ cup freshly squeezed orange juice
½ cup plain yogurt
1 large egg
½ tsp. almond extract
3 cups flour
4 tsp. baking powder
½ tsp. baking soda

¼ tsp. salt
1 stick butter, cut up
½ cup sugar
½ cup finely chopped blanched
   almonds
1½ Tbsp. freshly grated orange peel

Preheat oven to 375 degrees.

Grate the peel before juicing the orange! Measure juice then yogurt into a 2-cup glass measuring cup. Whisk in egg and almond extract until smooth. In large bowl, stir flour, baking powder, baking soda, and salt until mixed well; cut in butter until mixture looks like cornmeal. Add sugar, almonds, and orange peel. Toss to distribute evenly. Pour in egg mixture and gently stir with fork until soft dough forms. Turn out onto a lightly floured board and knead 10 times. Cut dough in half and form 2 separate discs about ½ inch thick. Cut each into 8 wedges and place on ungreased cookie sheet.

Bake about 25 minutes or until preferred brownness. Cool on wire rack.

Tip: Milk or buttermilk will also work nicely in place of plain yogurt.

Danish Breakfast Pastry

This recipe makes my husband crazy with its melt-in-your-mouth homemade goodness!

Pastry
- 1 cup flour
- 1 stick butter, cut into small cubes
- pinch of salt
- 2 Tbsp. water or more

Custard
- 1 stick butter, softened
- 1 cup flour
- pinch of salt
- 1 cup cold water
- 3 eggs

Icing
- 2 cups powdered sugar
- ½ tsp. almond extract
- milk

Using pastry cutter or food processor, cut butter into flour until you have a sandy consistency; add salt and blend in water a little at a time until dough is pliable. Spread very thin with fingers on large, lightly greased and floured cookie sheet. You should have about a 14×10 inch rectangle.

To make custard, melt butter in medium saucepan; whisk in flour and salt. Add water and cook, whisking until smooth and thick. Remove from heat and continue whisking in eggs one at a time. Spread custard over pastry, almost to edges, and bake at 400 degrees for 10 minutes. Lower heat to 350 degrees and bake about 35 minutes. Remove from oven.

Make icing. In medium bowl, whisk together powdered sugar, extract and enough milk to make a thin icing; drizzle over pastry while still warm and sprinkle with slivered or finely chopped almonds.

Holiday Sausage Bake

Serve with fresh fruit and buttered toast for a high protein brunch dish suitable for company.

  1 stick butter
  8 cups chopped fresh broccoli
  1 cup finely chopped onion
12 eggs
  2 cups whipping cream
  2 cups shredded cheddar cheese, divided
  1 lb. breakfast sausage, cooked, drained, and crumbled
  2 tsp. salt
  1 tsp. pepper

Preheat oven to 350 degrees.

Melt butter in skillet over medium heat; add broccoli and onion and sauté until tender, about 5 minutes. Set aside.

In a large bowl, beat eggs; add cream and 1½ cups of cheese. Mix well. Stir in sautéed broccoli and onion, prepared sausage, salt, and pepper. Pour into greased 3-quart casserole dish and set into a larger pan. Place in preheated oven and pour 1 inch of hot water into the outer pan. Bake uncovered at 350 degrees for 45–50 minutes or until knife inserted in center comes out clean.

Sprinkle with remaining ½ cup cheese and let stand for 10 minutes before serving.

Tip: Substitute 1 lb. of crispy fried bacon or 1 cup of chopped ham for sausage.

Huevos Ole

This breakfast serves a dozen friends—but it halves easily to feed 6. Warm corn or flour tortillas and salsa complete the dish!

1 dozen eggs, beaten
½ pint sour cream
1 lb. cubed ham
1 (32 oz.) can tomato pieces, well drained
1 green pepper, chopped
1 small onion, chopped
½ lb. shredded cheese
1 stick butter, melted
¼ tsp. salt
⅛ tsp. pepper

Mix all ingredients together in a large bowl and transfer to a 4-quart casserole dish. Bake at 350 degrees for 50 minutes.

Tip: For a spicier dish, switch tomato pieces with 2 (4 oz.) cans chopped green chilies and replace the chopped green bell pepper with a red one.

Lazy Morning French Toast

Make this up the night before for a wake-up treat!

  1 loaf crusty French bread
  1 (8 oz.) pkg. cream cheese, cubed
  1 stick butter, melted
2½ cups half and half
  ¼ cup maple syrup
  8 eggs

Cut bread into 1–2 inch chunky cubes. Sprinkle half evenly over the bottom of a 9×13 inch baking pan. Toss cream cheese pieces over bottom layer; top with remaining bread cubes.

In large bowl, mix melted butter, half and half, maple syrup, and eggs until creamy. It may look a bit curdled when the butter firms back up—just keep mixing until it's as smooth as you can get it. Pour over bread; press down to moisten. Cover; refrigerate overnight.

In the morning, remove cover and bake 50 minutes to an hour at 350 degrees. Serve hot.

Tips

If you'd like to jazz it up a bit, sprinkle a light layer of chopped nuts, raisins, or well-drained fresh fruit over the top of the cream cheese before adding the final layer of bread.

Top with a shake or two of cinnamon before baking.

Use flavored cream cheese like blueberry or strawberry in place of the plain variety.

Serve with hot maple syrup, butter, and toppings like toasted coconut, jams, or preserves—or even peanut butter!

Laid Back Butterhorns

Dough
- 4½ cups flour
- 3 Tbsp. sugar
- 1 cup cold butter, cut into small pieces
- 2 pkgs. yeast (4½ tsp. powdered yeast)
- ¼ cup warm water (100–110 degrees)
- 1 cup milk
- 3 eggs
- ⅓ cup sugar
- 1 Tbsp. cinnamon
- softened butter for spreading

Glaze
- ½ cup powdered sugar
- 2 tsp. milk
- ½ tsp. almond extract (or vanilla if preferred)

In small bowl, mix yeast with warm water to soften; set aside. In large mixing bowl, sift flour and add sugar; cut butter into sugar and flour mixture until the mixture resembles fine cornmeal. Make a well in the center of the pastry mixture; pour milk, eggs, and yeast mixture into the well. Mix thoroughly. Dough will be sticky and soft. Cover with plastic wrap and set in fridge overnight (or 8 hours) to rest.

After the dough has rested in the fridge, remove it and roll out on a lightly floured board or counter into a 9×12 rectangle, adding flour as necessary to keep from sticking. Combine ⅓ cup sugar and 1 Tbsp. cinnamon. Spread dough with softened butter and sprinkle with cinnamon and sugar mixture. Roll up like a jelly roll. Cut in ½-inch slices and place cut side up on greased cookie sheet. Lightly flatten butterhorns with palm of hand. Bake at 350 degrees for 10–15 minutes. Cool 10 minutes. While butterhorns are cooling make glaze. Mix well in a small bowl. Drizzle glaze on top and serve warm.

Sausage & Cheese Strudel

Filling
- 2 Tbsp. butter
- 2 Tbsp. flour
- 1 cup milk
- ½ cup shredded Swiss cheese
- 2 Tbsp. shredded Parmesan cheese
- ¼ tsp. salt
- ⅛ tsp. cayenne pepper
- ⅛ tsp. nutmeg
- ¼ lb. bulk pork sausages
- 5 large eggs, beaten
- 1½ tsp. thyme
- 1 Tbsp. chopped fresh parsley

Preheat oven to 375 degrees. Melt butter in small saucepan. Blend in flour and cook over medium heat until smooth and bubbly, about 1 minute. Gradually add milk; cook until mixture boils and thickens, stirring constantly. Boil 1 minute. Add Swiss and Parmesan cheeses, salt, cayenne pepper, and nutmeg. Stir until cheeses are melted. Set aside. In medium skillet, brown sausage, drain. Stir in eggs and thyme. Cook over medium heat until eggs are just set. Stir in cheese sauce and parsley. Cool completely.

(Continued on next page.)

Sausage & Cheese Strudel continued . . .

Pastry
- 5 frozen phyllo pastry sheets, thawed
- 1 stick butter, melted
- ¼ cup dry bread crumbs

Topping
- 1 Tbsp. shredded Parmesan cheese
- 2 Tbsp. chopped fresh parsley

Unroll phyllo sheets and cover with plastic wrap or towel. Brush 1 phyllo sheet with melted butter and sprinkle with bread crumbs. Fold in half lengthwise and brush with butter. Place ½ cup filling on bottom of short side of phyllo, leaving 1-inch edge on bottom and sides. Turn up edge, fold in sides, and roll up. Place seam-side-down on ungreased cookie sheet.

In a small bowl, combine topping ingredients. Brush strudel with melted butter and sprinkle with topping. Repeat with remaining phyllo sheets, filling, and topping. Bake at 375 degrees for 15 minutes or until crisp and light brown.

Yield: 5 servings, but can easily be doubled.

Cakes

Apricot Cake Deluxe
Oatmeal Gooey-Cake
Old-Fashioned Butter Cake
Snackin' Date Cake

Save your butter wrappers to grease pans. Just store in a plastic resealable baggie in the freezer until you need one. Easy!

Apricot Cake Deluxe

Try this recipe with applesauce or carrot baby food too!

Dough
- 3 eggs
- 2 cups sugar
- 1¼ cups vegetable oil
- 3 small jars apricot baby food
- 2 cups flour
- 2 tsp. cinnamon
- 1 tsp. baking soda
- 1 cup chopped pecans or walnuts

Icing
- 1 stick butter
- 1 (8 oz.) pkg. cream cheese
- 1 lb. powdered sugar
- 1 tsp. vanilla

Combine eggs, sugar, and oil; add baby food. Sift flour, cinnamon, and baking soda; add to wet mixture. Bake in a 12×9×2 inch pan at 350 degrees for 35 minutes or until done. Cool.

To make icing, blend ingredients together until smooth. Frost cooled cake.

Oatmeal Gooey-Cake

......Just like Grandma used to make! It's a perfect after school snack......

Dough

- 1 cup oatmeal (not instant!)
- 1¼ cups boiling water
- 1 stick butter
- 1 egg
- 1 tsp. cinnamon
- 1 cup white sugar
- 1 cup brown sugar
- 1½ cup flour
- 1 tsp. soda

Frosting

- ½ stick butter
- ½ cup brown sugar
- ¼ cup cream
- 1 cup coconut
- 1 tsp. vanilla

Cream oatmeal, water, and butter; beat in egg. Mix all dry ingredients together and slowly blend into oatmeal batter. Pour into greased and floured 9×13 pan and bake at 350 degrees for 25–30 minutes.

Make frosting by combining butter, sugar, and cream in sauce pan. Cook until thick; remove from heat and add coconut and vanilla. Frost cooled cake.

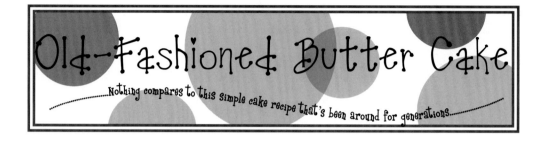

Old-Fashioned Butter Cake

Nothing compares to this simple cake recipe that's been around for generations...

1 stick butter
1 cup sugar
2 eggs
⅔ cup milk
2 cups sifted flour
1 Tbsp. baking powder
¼ tsp. salt
1 tsp. vanilla

Cream butter and add sugar gradually; blend thoroughly. Add eggs ,beating well. Sift flour, salt, and baking powder. Combine flour mixture with creamed mixture, adding milk alternately. Add vanilla. Bake in two greased 8-inch layer pans at 375 degrees for 25 minutes or until done.

Tip: I've come to appreciate the value of a parchment paper lined pan—you'll never worry about cakes getting stuck to the bottom again!

Snackin' Date Cake

This cake is rich and full of "grandma memories." Very tasty for the holidays!

Dough

  1½ cups flour
  ½ tsp. cinnamon
  ½ tsp. cloves
  1 tsp. baking soda
  1 stick butter, softened
  1 cup brown sugar
  1 cup sour milk or buttermilk
  1 egg, beaten
  1 cup chopped dates
  ½ cup chopped walnuts

Caramel Glaze

  ½ cup sugar
  ¼ cup buttermilk
  ¼ tsp. baking soda
  1 Tbsp. white corn syrup
  ½ stick butter
  ½ tsp. vanilla

Sift together flour, cinnamon, cloves, and baking soda; set aside. Cream butter and brown sugar; mix in egg, then brown sugar. Beat in buttermilk and flour mixture alternately; mix in dates and walnuts by hand.

Pour batter into lightly greased and floured 9×9 inch pan. Bake at 350 degrees for 25–30 minutes or until toothpick comes out clean.

Make glaze 20 minutes before cake is ready. Bring the ingredients to a slow boil in a saucepan stirring constantly. Pour over hot cake.

Tip: Delicious served with fresh whipped cream.

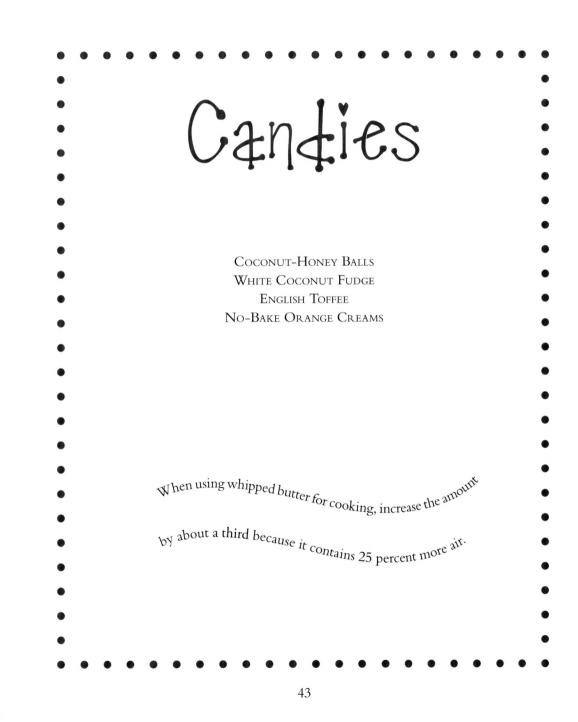

Candies

Coconut-Honey Balls
White Coconut Fudge
English Toffee
No-Bake Orange Creams

When using whipped butter for cooking, increase the amount by about a third because it contains 25 percent more air.

Coconut-Honey Balls

1 stick butter
2 Tbsp. milk
1 cup flour
¾ cup honey
¼ tsp. salt
1 cup coconut
1 tsp. vanilla
2 cups rice cereal (like Rice Krispies)

Combine all ingredients except vanilla and cereal in saucepan. Cook over medium heat, stirring constantly, until dough leaves sides of pan and forms a ball, about 7–10 minutes. Remove from heat, cool slightly, and add vanilla; stir well. Carefully stir in cereal; shape into 1-inch balls. Roll in additional coconut if desired. Store in refrigerator.

Yield: 3 dozen.

Tip: If you'd like to have a finer coconut coating, run your toasted coconut through a food grinder or processor before rolling honey balls around in it. An extra step that gives more of a professional look!

White Coconut Fudge

Friends and co-workers will love this as a holiday gift... ...Just make sure to make a second batch for your own family!

     4 cups sugar
 1¼ cups evaporated milk
     1 stick butter, cut into small pieces
     1 tsp. vanilla
 1–2 cups toasted coconut
     1 cup chopped nuts

In medium size saucepan, cook sugar and milk over medium to medium high heat until it boils; boil 6 minutes.

Remove from heat and stir in butter, vanilla, coconut, and nuts. Cool to room temperature and pour into a 9×13 inch greased pan to set.

Tip: To toast coconut, spread shredded, sweetened coconut on baking sheet in a thin layer. Bake in a preheated 350 degree oven, stirring about every minute until you reach the desired light brown color, usually no more then 5 minutes.

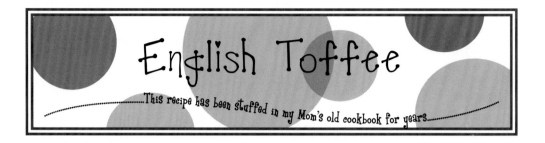

English Toffee

...This recipe has been stuffed in my Mom's old cookbook for years...

1½ stick butter, melted
1 cup sugar
¾ cup blanched almonds, chopped
1 cup chopped pecans
5 (1.55 oz.) Hershey's milk chocolate bars

Combine all ingredients except pecans and chocolate bars in saucepan. Cook, stirring constantly and rapidly, until mixture starts to smoke.

Pour immediately onto buttered cookie sheet and spread as thin as possible. Place chocolate bars on top and, when melted, spread evenly over candy and sprinkle with pecans. Press nuts into chocolate; cool and break into pieces.

No-Bake Orange Creams

...These little miracles are soft, flavorful, and delightfully rich!...

1 lb. vanilla wafers, crushed
1 lb. powdered sugar
1 stick butter, melted
1 (12 oz.) can frozen orange juice, thawed but not diluted
   finely chopped nuts or coconut

Mix wafers, powdered sugar, melted butter, and orange juice together. Form 2-inch balls out of dough by rolling in palm of hands; roll in nuts or coconut. Place on wax paper lined cookie sheet, cover lightly with plastic wrap and chill to firm. Store in fridge.

Yield: 3 dozen.

Tip: If you use only 6 oz. of orange juice, these will harden and keep for a long time.

Cookies

Cookie Pops
Apricot Streusel Bars
Choco-nana Bonanza Bars
Pecan Pie Bites
Pecan Snowballs

Salt content in butter can vary so much that I always recommend using unsalted or sweet butter to bake with and regular butter for savory kitchen dishes.

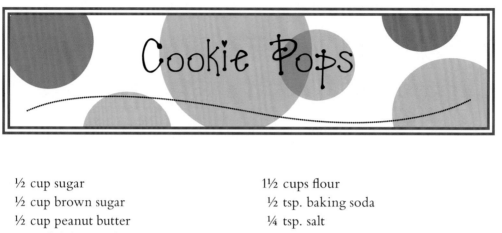

Cookie Pops

½ cup sugar
½ cup brown sugar
½ cup peanut butter
1 stick butter, softened
1 tsp. vanilla
1 egg

1½ cups flour
½ tsp. baking soda
¼ tsp. salt
10–15 popsicle sticks
1 bag fun size Milky Way or Snickers bars

Preheat to 350 degrees.

Combine sugars, peanut butter, butter, vanilla, and egg. Sift flour, baking soda, and salt together, then mix into margarine blend. Put sticks into small ends of candy bars. Shape dough around bars, completely covering candy. Bake 4 inches apart 14–16 minutes or until golden brown. Cool completely and remove.

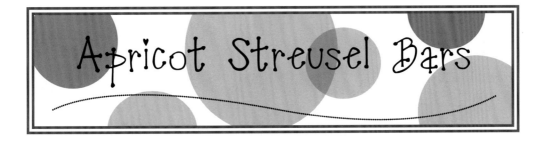

Apricot Streusel Bars

½ cup powdered sugar
½ cup finely chopped almonds
1¾ cups flour
¼ tsp. salt
1½ sticks butter
¼ tsp. almond extract
12 oz. apricot preserves
2 Tbsp. brown sugar
¼ tsp. cinnamon

In food processor, pulse dry ingredients until well blended. Cut butter into small pieces and add to processor along with almond extract. Blend together in processor until the mixture has a sandy consistency. Press onto bottom of lightly greased 9×13 inch pan; reserve 1 cup for topping.

Place preserves in small bowl and microwave to loosen. Spread evenly over prepared crust when slightly warm.

Using food processor, pulse brown sugar and cinnamon into reserved topping; sprinkle over top of preserves. Bake 30 minutes in a 350 degree oven. Cut bars while still warm.

Tip: Delicious with strawberry preserves too!

Choco-nana Bonanza Bars

1 stick butter, softened
1 cup sugar
1 egg
1 tsp. vanilla
1½ cups mashed bananas
1½ cups flour
1 tsp. baking powder
1 tsp. baking soda
½ tsp. salt
¼ cup cocoa
⅓ cup chopped walnuts or pecans
⅓ cup peanut butter chips

Cream butter and sugar until well blended. Beat in the egg and vanilla. Blend in the mashed banana. In separate bowl, combine flour, baking powder, baking soda, and salt; add to creamed mixture. Divide batter in half. Add cocoa to *one half of batter.*

Spread cocoa batter mixture in greased 9×13 inch pan. Sprinkle evenly with nuts and chocolate chips and top with remaining half of batter, spreading carefully. Bake at 350 degrees for 25 minutes.

Tip: Top with powdered sugar icing if desired.

Pecan Pie Bites

Crust
- 1 (3 oz.) pkg. cream cheese
- 1 stick butter
- 1 cup sifted flour

Pecan Filling
- 1 egg
- ¾ cup brown sugar
- 1 Tbsp. soft butter
- 1 tsp. vanilla
- dash of salt
- ⅔ cup finely chopped pecans

Let cream cheese and butter soften to room temperature. Blend together then stir in flour and wrap tightly in plastic wrap; chill for about 1 hour. Shape into 2 dozen 1-inch balls. Place in ungreased 1¾ inch muffin tins, press dough against bottom and sides.

Preheat oven to 375 degrees.

Beat together egg, brown sugar, butter, vanilla, and salt, just until smooth. Sprinkle a few pecans in bottom of pastry cups. Add egg mixture and top with more pecan pieces (you may not need to use them all). Bake for 25 minutes or until filling is set. Cool and remove from pan.

Tip: Have you ever used a wooden tamper to shape your dough balls to mini muffin cups? I just dip the tamper in sugar before pressing it onto the dough for easy release.

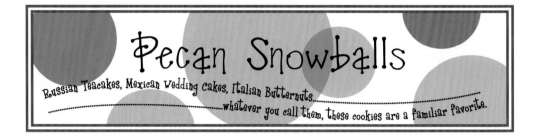

Pecan Snowballs

Russian Teacakes, Mexican Wedding cakes, Italian Butternuts...

...whatever you call them, these cookies are a familiar favorite.

  2 sticks butter, softened
½ cup powdered sugar
½ tsp. vanilla
1¾ cups flour
½ cup finely chopped pecans or walnuts
    powdered sugar

Cream butter and sugar together *slowly* . . . or else you'll get a little unexpected face powder! Then beat until light and fluffy. Add vanilla and then slowly add flour. Mix in nuts. Chill dough for at least 2 hours. Form into 1-inch balls, place on cookie sheet. Bake at 350 degrees for 20 minutes. Roll in powdered sugar while still warm.

Yield: 4 dozen.

Desserts

Bob's Hot Fudge Sauce

Blueberry Cream Pie

Brown Sugar Squares
with Orange Icing

Chocolate "Is My Friend" Indulgence

Cranberry Walnut Pie

Cranberry Cream Yummies

Cream Puff Pudding Bake

Diana's Peach Cobbler

Fudge Pie

Graham Cracker Walnut Pie Crust

Lemon-Lime Delight Bars

Luscious Berry Cream Pastry

Peanut Butter Cups

Praline Ice Cream Dreams

To brown butter for sauces, melt slowly so that it browns evenly without burning. Be careful—burnt butter tastes bitter!

Bob's Hot Fudge Sauce

.......One of the nicest salesmen I've ever known sold me on his fabulous fudge sauce.......

  1 pkg. semi-sweet chocolate chips
  2 sticks butter
2⅔ cups evaporated milk
  4 cups powdered sugar
  2 tsp. vanilla

Melt chocolate chips and butter in pan over medium heat. Gradually stir in evaporated milk and sugar; bring to boil. Boil and stir constantly for 8 minutes. Remove from heat and add vanilla.

Blueberry Cream Pie

Impressive! Delightful! Encore!

Crust
- 1 cup flour
- 1 stick butter
- ½ cup chopped walnuts

Center
- 1 (8 oz.) pkg. cream cheese, softened
- 2 Tbsp. half and half
- ¼ cup powdered sugar
- 1 tsp. lemon zest

Filling
- 4 cups fresh blueberries
- 1 Tbsp. lemon juice
- 2½ Tbsp. cornstarch
- 1 cup (or less) sugar

To make crust, cut butter into flour until it has the consistency of cornmeal; mix in walnuts. Press into 9-inch pie plate. Bake at 350 degrees until light golden, about 15 minutes. Chill.

To make center, whip together ingredients and spread on cooled crust. Stick the pie back in the fridge.

To make filling, mash enough berries into ¼ cup water to make 1½ cups. Pour into saucepan and mix in sugar and cornstarch. Bring to a boil, stirring frequently until thickened. Remove from heat and gently stir in remaining berries. Chill well. Spread over crust and center.

Top with whipped cream before serving.

Brown Sugar Squares
with Orange Icing

Dough
- 1 cup flour
- 2 Tbsp. brown sugar
- 1 stick butter
- 2 eggs, beaten
- 1½ cups brown sugar
- 1 tsp. vanilla
- ½ cup chopped walnuts or pecans
- ½ cup coconut
- 2 Tbsp. flour
- ½ tsp. salt

Orange Icing
- 1 cup powdered sugar
- 2 Tbsp. butter, melted
- orange juice

Mix flour and 2 Tbsp. brown sugar; cut in butter like a pie crust. Press into the bottom of a 9×13 pan. Bake 12–15 minutes in 350 degree oven.

Combine remaining ingredients and spread on baked crust. Bake 30 minutes at 350 degrees. Cool.

To make icing, mix sugar and butter with enough orange juice to spread. Frost cooled cake.

Chocolate "Is My Friend" Indulgence

Replace the chocolate pudding with pistachio if you'd rather...

1 cup flour
½ cup coarsely chopped walnuts
1 stick butter, softened
1 (8 oz.) pkg. cream cheese, softened
1 cup powdered sugar
1 (16 oz.) container whipped topping (like Cool Whip)
2 small pkgs. instant chocolate pudding
3 cups milk

Cut butter into flour; blend in walnuts. Spread in bottom of 9×13 pan and bake for 20 minutes at 350 degrees. Cool.

Blend cream cheese and sugar together with fork. Add half of whipped topping and continue to mix. Spread evenly onto cooled crust.

Whisk pudding and milk together until well blended and spread over cream cheese mixture. Your final layer is the remaining whipped topping. Sprinkle with more nuts if desired and chill.

Yield: Serves a dozen . . . or maybe just 4 really happy adults!

Cranberry Walnut Pie

So simple . . . yet so delicious. Serve warm with vanilla bean ice cream!

    2 cups fresh or frozen cranberries
  ½ cup chopped walnuts
1½ cups sugar, divided
    1 stick butter
    1 cup flour
    1 tsp. almond extract
    2 eggs, beaten

Lightly grease 10-inch pie pan; cover bottom with cranberries and nuts. Sprinkle with ½ cup sugar. In large bowl, melt butter; add flour, almond extract, remaining sugar, and eggs. Mix well and pour over cranberries and nuts.

Bake at 350 degrees for 35–40 minutes or until knife comes out clean.

Cranberry Cream Yummies

Who says cranberries have to wait until the holidays to come out of the cupboard?

Crust
- 1 cup flour
- 1 stick butter
- ⅓ cup sugar

Filling
- 1 (8 oz.) pkg. cream cheese, room temperature
- 1 egg
- 1 tsp. vanilla
- ⅓ cup sugar
- 1 (16 oz.) can jellied cranberries

Preheat oven to 350 degrees.

Mix flour and sugar, then cut in butter with pastry blender until mixture resembles coarse crumbs. Press into bottom of 7×11-inch pan. Bake 20 minutes until brown. Cool.

To make filling, beat cream cheese, egg, vanilla, and sugar until smooth. Make a layer of jellied cranberries over crust and pour cream cheese mixture over the top. Bake 30–35 minutes until toothpick comes out clean.

Cool and cut into squares.

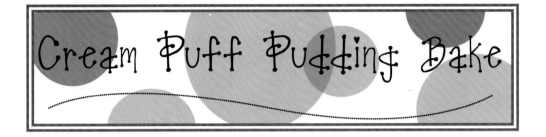
Cream Puff Pudding Bake

1 stick butter
1 cup water
1 cup flour
1 large vanilla instant pudding
2½ cups milk
1 (8 oz.) pkg. cream cheese
1 (8 oz.) container non-dairy whipped topping (like Cool Whip)
½ cup chocolate chips
2 Tbsp. butter
3 Tbsp. milk
1 cup powdered sugar

For the crust, boil 1 stick butter and 1 cup water; remove from heat. Add flour; stir until it forms a ball. Beat in 4 eggs, one at a time. Spread in greased 9×13 pan. Bake at 400 degrees for 30 minutes. Cool.

With electric mixer, blend pudding, milk, and cream cheese together until smooth. Pour over cooled puff. Spread Cool Whip over pudding. Chill.

For topping; melt chocolate chips, butter and milk in double boiler; remove from heat. Mix in powdered sugar until smooth and cool to room temperature. Drizzle over top with spoon and chill before serving.

Tip: Try swirling jam or preserves into pudding mixture before topping with Cool Whip.

Diana's Peach Cobbler

    1 stick butter, melted
    1 cup sugar
    1 cup flour
 2½ tsp. baking powder
    ¾ cup milk
    6 peaches, sliced

Pour melted butter in 9×13 pan. Mix together sugar, flour, baking powder and milk. Pour over butter—*do not stir.* Place sliced peaches over top and bake at 350 degrees for 40–45 minutes. Serve warm with ice cream.

Tip: Try sprinkling cinnamon or nutmeg over top of dough before placing peaches in pan.

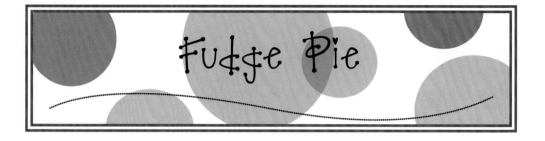

Fudge Pie

2 (1 oz.) squares unsweetened chocolate
1 stick butter
1 cup sugar
¼ cup flour
2 eggs, beaten
1 tsp. vanilla

Melt chocolate and butter in double boiler; remove from heat. Sift together sugar and flour; add to chocolate mixture. Whisk in eggs and vanilla. Pour into buttered 9-inch pie pan and bake 20 minutes at 350 degrees. Serve hot with ice cream.

Tip: Can be made early and heated for serving.

Graham Cracker Walnut Pie Crust

  2 cups graham cracker crumbs
½ tsp. salt
  1 stick butter, melted
  1 cup finely chopped nuts
¼ cup honey

Mix all together. Press into pie pan and bake at 375 degrees for 5–7 minutes. Cool before adding filling.

Yield: 2 pie crusts.

Suggested fillings

Key Lime
Banana Cream
Coconut Cream

Lemon-Lime Delight Bars

Throw a few of these bars into a blender with some vanilla ice cream. You'll have a refreshing shake with cookie bits!

  2 sticks butter
½ cup powdered sugar
  2 cups flour
  4 eggs, beaten
  2 cups sugar
¼ cup flour
  4 Tbsp. fresh lemon juice
  2 Tbsp. fresh lime juice & zest to taste

Combine butter, powdered sugar, and flour, mixing well. Press into 9×13 pan and bake 15 minutes at 350 degrees.

Blend eggs, sugar, flour, juices, and zest together; pour into slightly cooled crust. Bake at 350 degrees for 25 minutes or until set.

Chill and sprinkle with additional powdered sugar if desired.

Luscious Berry Cream Pastry

Showcase summer's best fruits!

1 (18.25 oz) box yellow cake mix
1 stick butter
½ cup coconut
3 cups berries, rinsed and cleaned
2 Tbsp. sugar
½ tsp. cinnamon
1 egg, slightly beaten
1 cup sour cream

Cut together cake mix, butter, and coconut. Press into the bottom and half an inch up the sides of a 9×13 pan. Bake at 350 degrees for 10 minutes. Remove from oven and arrange fruit over the crust, sprinkle with sugar and cinnamon.

Whisk egg and sour cream together and spread on top to within half inch of edge (not all the way to edge so you can check color of crust as it bakes). Bake 15 more minutes or until crust is a delicate brown. Cool just until warm and cut into squares to serve.

Tip: Blackberries are my favorite in this, but thinly sliced peaches are also a perfect match.

Peanut Butter Cups

  2 sticks butter
  1 cup peanut butter
1¾ cups crushed graham crackers
  2 cups powdered sugar
  2 cups chocolate chips

Melt butter and peanut butter together. Stir in powdered sugar, then crackers. Line 13×9 inch pan with parchment paper and press mixture firmly into bottom of pan; place in refrigerator for about 15 minutes.

Melt chocolate chips in double boiler or microwave. Remove peanut butter mixture from refrigerator and spread chocolate on top. Chill until firm and remove from fridge. Cut into squares when softened to room temperature.

Praline Ice Cream Dreams

Go a little bananas and make your own tropical caramel sauce and replace the pecans with macadamia nuts! Recipe included!

Ice Cream
- ½ cup brown sugar
- ½ cup oatmeal
- 2 cups flour
- 1 cup chopped pecans
- 2 sticks butter, melted
- ½ tsp. salt
- 1½ (12.2 oz.) jars caramel ice cream topping
- ½ gallon vanilla ice cream, softened

Homemade topping
- 1 stick butter
- 1 cup brown sugar
- 1 tsp. orange zest
- ½ cup pineapple juice
- 4 tsp. vanilla extract
- 3 small ripe bananas, sliced

Mix brown sugar, oatmeal, flour, and chopped nuts together with melted butter and salt. Mix like cookie dough; spread on foil-lined cookie sheet. Bake 10–12 minutes at 400 degrees. Crumble while still hot. Place half of the oatmeal crumbs into the bottom of a 9×13 pan. Pour half jar of caramel topping over crumbs. Spread ice cream over caramel. Cover with reserved crumbs and drizzle with another jar of caramel. Freeze and cut into squares before serving.

To make topping, melt butter, in large skillet over medium heat; stir in sugar, add orange zest, and mix well. Mixture will start to simmer; when you begin to see crystallization, add juice and continue to stir until thickened to desired consistency. Remove from heat and add bananas, folding them into caramel so they'll keep their shape. Carefully blend in vanilla. Cool before drizzling over ice cream.

Main Dishes

Beefed up Man's Meal
Almond Chicken Casserole
Cheese Lovers' Chicken Fettuccine
Cheesy Linguine Tart
Chicken & Wild Rice Bake
Chicken Dijon in Phyllo
Creamy Chicken Bake
Crepes Ensenada
Garlic Parmesan Chicken
Green Chicken Casserole
Grilled Crab & Cheddar Sammy

Honey Mustard Chicken for a Crowd
Kentucky Hot Browns
Ramen-Topped Oriental Salad
Reuben Bake
Ritzy Chicken Casserole
Shrimp Enchiladas
Spinach Enchilada Casserole
Stuffed Pork Chops
Swiss Chicken Bliss
Tuna Bake
Wednesday Night Stroganoff

Keep butter from burning when frying by mixing in a small amount of oil or shortening . . . some say a mixture of half and half works best.

Beefed-up Man's Meal

Meat

1 (2 ½ lb.) boneless
   chuck roast, cut into
   1 inch cubes
2 large onions, chopped
2 Tbsp. butter
2 Tbsp. vegetable oil
1 (8 oz.) can tomato
   sauce
2 tsp. sugar

2 tsp. paprika
2 tsp. Worcestershire
   sauce
1 tsp. salt
1½ tsp. caraway seeds
1 tsp. dill weed
¼ tsp. pepper
⅛ tsp. garlic powder
1 cup sour cream

Garlic Toast

½ stick butter, softened
1 tsp. garlic powder
   french bread

Place butter and oil in large saucepan or Dutch Oven over medium high heat. Once butter has melted, add cubed beef and onions. Sauté until meat is browned and onion is soft. In a separate bowl, mix up the rest of the ingredients except sour cream.

Pour over browned meat in pan; bring to boil and reduce heat. Cover and simmer for 2 hours or until meat is tender. Remove from heat and stir in sour cream. While meat is cooking, make garlic butter and set aside. Approximately 30 minutes before meat is done, toast 10–12 thick sliced French bread; cool slightly and spread with garlic butter on one side. Place in 250-degree oven until serving time.

Stir 2 Tbsp. butter into your choice of hot cooked egg noodles, mashed potatoes, or steamed rice and serve meat on top. Whip up a green salad and serve the garlic toast!

Yield: 4–6 servings.

Almond Chicken Casserole

Superb served with steamed rice and fresh peas

    4 cups chicken breasts, cooked and chopped
    1 (10.75 oz.) can cream of chicken soup
    1 (8 oz.) container sour cream
 1½ cups Chow Mein Noodles
    4 oz. slivered almonds
    1 stick butter

Mix the chicken, soup, and sour cream together in large bowl. Pour into a lightly greased 9×13 casserole dish; sprinkle Chow Mein Noodles over top, then almonds. Dot with pats of butter. Bake at 350 degrees for 30 minutes.

Yield: 4 servings.

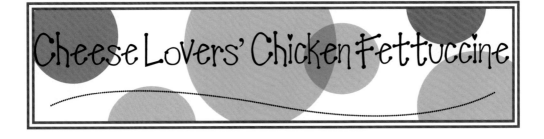
Cheese Lovers' Chicken Fettuccine

Fettuccine

8 oz. fettuccine, cooked al dente and drained
1 (10.75 oz.) can mushroom soup
1 (8 oz.) pkg. cream cheese
10 medium fresh mushrooms, sliced
1 cup half and half
1 stick butter
1 tsp. fresh crushed garlic
¾ cup Parmesan cheese
½ cup shredded mozzarella cheese
½ cup shredded Swiss cheese
2½ cups cubed chicken

Topping

⅓ cup seasoned bread crumbs
2 Tbsp. butter, melted
1½ Tbsp. Parmesan cheese

In large saucepan, combine soup, cream cheese, mushrooms, half and half, butter and crushed garlic. Stir in cheeses; cook over low heat until melted, stirring frequently. Add chicken. Heat through. Add cooked fettuccine to sauce. Transfer to 2½-quart baking dish. Combine topping ingredients and sprinkle over chicken mixture. Cover and bake at 350 degrees for 20–25 minutes or until topping is golden brown.

Yield: 6–8 servings.

Tip: If preferred, sauté mixed chopped veggies and add to sauce for additional flavor and coloring. Delicious with shrimp, clams, or bay scallops added in as well!

Cheesy Linguine Tart

1 stick butter, divided
2 cloves garlic, minced
30 thin French bread slices
3 Tbsp. flour
1 tsp. salt
¼ tsp. white pepper
   dash of nutmeg
2½ cups milk
¼ cup shredded Parmesan cheese

2 eggs, beaten
8 oz. Fresh linguine, cooked and
   drained
2 cups shredded mozzarella cheese
⅓ cup sliced green onions
2 Tbsp. minced fresh basil
2 plum tomatoes, each cut lengthwise
   into eighths

Preheat oven to 400 degrees.

Melt ½ stick butter in small saucepan over medium heat. Add garlic; cook 1 minute. Brush 10-inch pie plate with butter mixture. Line bottom and side of pie plate with bread, allowing a 1-inch overhang. Brush bread with remaining butter mixture. Bake 5 minutes or until lightly browned.

Melt remaining ½ stick butter in medium saucepan over low heat. Stir in flour and seasonings. Gradually stir in milk; cook, stirring constantly, until thickened. Add Parmesan cheese. Stir some of the sauce into eggs; stir back into sauce. Set aside.

Lower oven temperature to 350 degrees. Combine linguine, 1¼ cups mozzarella cheese, onions, and basil in large bowl. Pour sauce over linguine mixture; toss to coat. Pour into "pie crust" and arrange tomatoes on top; sprinkle with remaining ¾ cup mozzarella cheese. Bake 25 minutes or until warm; let stand 5 minutes.

Chicken & Wild Rice Bake

1 cup uncooked wild rice
½ cup chopped onion
8 oz. fresh, sliced mushrooms
1 stick butter
¼ cup flour
1½ cups chicken broth
1½ cup half and half
3 cups diced cooked chicken
¼ cup diced pimiento
2 Tbsp. snipped parsley
1½ tsp. salt
¼ tsp. pepper
½ cup toasted pine nuts

Prepare wild rice according to package directions; set aside. Cook chopped onion and mushrooms in butter until tender but not brown. Remove from heat; stir in flour. Add chicken broth to flour mixture, then add half and half. Cook and stir until mixture thickens.

Add wild rice, chicken, pimiento, parsley, salt, and pepper to thickened liquid. Place in a 2-quart casserole. Sprinkle with pine nuts. Bake at 350 degrees for 25–30 minutes or until hot.

Yield: 8 servings.

Chicken Dijon in Phyllo

3 whole chicken breasts, skinned and boned
½ tsp. salt
¼ tsp. white pepper
½ stick butter
½ cup Dijon mustard

2 cups heavy cream
8 phyllo pastry sheets
1½ stick butter, melted
¼ cup dry bread crumbs
1 egg
1 tsp. water

Cut chicken into 1-inch strips. Sprinkle with salt and pepper. In skillet, sauté chicken in ½ stick butter until no longer pink inside, about five minutes. Transfer to platter and keep warm.

Place mustard in skillet; whisk in cream until well blended. Reduce heat and simmer sauce until slightly thickened and reduced. Stir in any juices from chicken, then strain sauce as you pour over chicken.

Lay one sheet of phyllo on a damp dish towel, brush liberally with melted butter and sprinkle with bread crumbs. Layer 6 more phyllo sheets on top, preparing each with butter and bread crumbs. Top with last phyllo sheet, brushing only the borders with melted butter. Arrange chicken on lower third of long side of dough, leaving a 2-inch border along outside edges. Fold outside edges inward partially enclosing chicken, then roll up jelly-roll fashion. Place seam side down on lightly greased baking sheet. Beat egg with water and brush over dough to glaze. Bake at 450 degrees until phyllo is crisp and golden, 12–15 minutes. Cut into 2-inch slices and serve.

Creamy Chicken Bake

    1 stick butter
 ¼ cup flour
    2 cups broth
    1 cup half and half
    3 beaten eggs
    1 can cream of mushroom soup
 ½ cup chopped red or green bell peppers
    3 cups cooked and cubed chicken (or turkey)
       salt and pepper to taste
       buttered corn flakes

Blend butter and flour over low heat. Add broth and cream. When it begins to thicken, slowly add eggs. Add mushroom soup, peppers, chicken, salt, and pepper. Place in lightly greased 9×13 pan and cover with buttered corn flakes. Bake 30 minutes at 350 degrees.

Tip: To butter corn flakes, drizzle or lightly coat desired amount of butter on bowl of corn flakes and mix gently.

Crepes Ensenada

Crepes

- 12 flour tortillas
- 12 thin slices ham
- 1 lb. Jack cheese cut into 12 pieces
- 1 (7 oz.) can green chilies (seeded and cut into 12 strips)

Cheese Sauce

- 1 stick butter
- flour to thicken
- 4 cups milk
- ¾ lb. cheddar cheese, shredded
- 1 tsp. prepared mustard
- ½ tsp. salt
- paprika

Place ham, cheese, and chili on each tortilla; fold in sides then roll. Place in greased baking dish.

To make cheese sauce, melt butter and blend in flour; add remaining ingredients except paprika. Cook until smooth.

Pour cheese sauce over "crepes" to cover. Sprinkle with paprika and bake at 350 degrees for 45 minutes.

Garlic Parmesan Chicken

16 chicken tender strips
1 egg
2 Tbsp. milk
1 cup instant mashed potato flakes
1 tsp. Italian seasoning
1 Tbsp. crushed garlic
¼ cup shredded Parmesan cheese
1½ sticks butter

Beat egg and milk in bowl. In another bowl, mix potato flakes, Italian seasoning, garlic and Parmesan cheese. First roll the chicken in the egg mixture, then dredge in potato mixture. Place butter in shallow pan and put in hot oven until melted. Remove pan from oven, then roll coated chicken in butter, and place in the pan. Bake at 400 degrees for 30 minutes or until juices run clear and crust is brown.

Green Chicken Casserole

A pretty presentation caps off this divine dinner dish

1 cup broad, flat green noodles
1 large ripe avocado, peeled and sliced
2 Tbsp. fresh lime juice
1 stick butter
¼ cup flour
1 tsp. salt

5 dashes Tabasco
2¼ cups half and half
1 cup shredded cheddar cheese
6 (6 oz.) boneless, skinless chicken breast halves, poached
2 (4 oz.) cans chopped green chilies

Prepare noodles according to package directions; drain and set aside.

Preheat oven to 350 degrees. Drizzle avocado slices with lime juice and set aside.

Melt butter in 2-quart saucepan over low heat. Stir in flour, salt, and Tabasco, continuing to stir and cook over low heat until mixture bubbles.

Add half and half slowly, stirring constantly until mixture thickens; remove from heat. Add the cheese and stir until it melts. Reserve 1 cup of sauce; pour remaining sauce over cooked noodles, mixing well.

Place chicken in bottom of a 9×13×3 baking dish. Cover the chicken with the chopped green chilies. Spoon noodle mixture over all. Place avocado slices on top and pour reserved sauce over avocados. Bake uncovered for 35 minutes.

Yield: 6 servings.

Tip: To poach chicken breasts, add pieces to pot and barely cover with liquid. Cover and simmer over low heat until done, about 8–10 minutes. You can use chicken broth in place of water and add herbs or diced onions, carrots, celery, etc.

Grilled Crab & Cheddar Sammy

......Delicious served with seashell pasta salad......

½ cup mayonnaise
½ cup chili sauce
1 cup fresh crab, picked over to clean
4 cups shredded medium cheddar cheese
¼ cup chopped green olives
¼ cup chopped green onions
¼ cup chopped bell pepper
¼ cup chopped celery
12 slices sourdough bread
1 stick butter, melted

In medium bowl, stir together mayonnaise, chili sauce, and crabmeat. Add cheese, olives, onion, pepper and celery; mix thoroughly. Divide the filling between 6 slices of bread and top with remaining slices. Brush the top side with melted butter. Place in frying pan and brown over low heat, buttered side down, until cheese melts. Brush remaining side with melted butter, turn and continue to cook until both sides are golden brown.

Yield: 6 sandwiches.

Honey Mustard Chicken
for a Crowd

8 boneless, skinless chicken breasts
1 stick butter
½ cup honey
¼ cup Dijon mustard
1 tsp. curry powder
½ tsp. salt

Place chicken in a large, shallow baking pan. In saucepan, melt butter; stir in remaining ingredients and heat through. Brush glaze over chicken. Bake at 350 degrees for 1 hour 15 minutes or until chicken is golden brown. Baste with sauce frequently while baking. Delicious over brown butter pasta!

Kentucky Hot Browns

    1 lb. bacon, fried crisp
  16 pieces of bread
       turkey or chicken slices
    1 stick butter
    1 lb. shredded sharp cheddar cheese
    2 (5.5 oz.) cans evaporated milk
    2 cans mushroom soup, undiluted
  16 slices tomato

Toast slices of bread. Warm slices of turkey or chicken. Combine in saucepan the butter, cheese, milk, and soup. Heat until cheese melts.

Place toast on bottom of baking pan; top with warmed turkey or chicken slices. Cover with layers of tomatoes and a layer of bacon. Pour cheese sauce over all and broil until hot.

Ramen-Topped Oriental Salad

 1 stick butter
¼ cup sesame seeds
½ cup sunflower seeds
¼ cup slivered almonds
 2 pkgs. ramen noodles
¾ cup sugar
½ cup oil
½ cup cider vinegar

1½ Tbsp. soy sauce
 1 bunch of green onions, thinly sliced
 1 (8 oz.) can of water chestnuts,
    coarsely chopped
 1 cup loosely packed bean sprouts
 1 pkg. cole slaw mix
    shredded chicken or cooked shrimp

Melt butter in skillet and toast seeds, nuts, and ramen noodles until lightly browned (you can discard flavor pack from noodles). Drain and cool.

Mix sugar, oil, vinegar, and soy sauce together and heat in microwave to melt sugar, stirring often. Set aside to cool.

Mix green onions, sprouts, water chestnuts, cole slaw, and chicken or shrimp together in large bowl. Add salad dressing to taste. Serve on chilled plate topped with seed/nut mixture.

Tip: Top with drained mandarin oranges for a delicious addition.

Reuben Bake

  1 stick butter
  6 slices rye bread, cut into ½-inch cubes
  1 (32 oz.) jar sauerkraut, drained very well
  1 cup chopped onion
½ cup snipped fresh parsley
  2 tsp. caraway seeds
  4 cups shredded Swiss cheese
1⅓ cups Thousand Island salad dressing
  1 lb. thinly sliced cooked corned beef, coarsely chopped (from the deli)

In a large skillet, melt the butter over low heat. Add bread cubes and stir until coated. Remove from heat and set aside.

In a large bowl, combine drained sauerkraut, onion, parsley, and caraway seeds. Spread mixture evenly into an ungreased 13×9 pan. Layer with half the cheese, half the salad dressing, and all of the corned beef. Spread with remaining salad dressing and top off with remaining cheese. Sprinkle bread cubes over the top of the casserole.

Bake at 375 degrees for 35 minutes or until heated through and bread cubes are browned.

Yield: 6–8 servings.

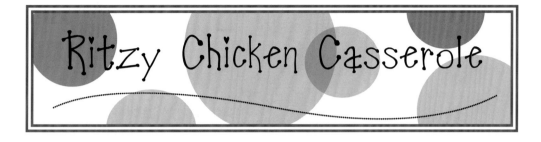

Ritzy Chicken Casserole

    1 (4 lb.) chicken
2–3 cloves garlic, chopped
    3 cups egg noodles
    4 cups chicken broth
    ½ cup flour
    ½ lb. shredded sharp cheddar cheese
    1 small box butter crackers (like Ritz crackers)
    1 stick butter, melted

Cover chicken with water in large saucepan; add garlic and preferred seasonings. Stew until tender; drain and cube. Cook noodles in salt water and drain. Thicken broth with flour. Mix all together; add cheese and pour into greased 9×13 pan. Crush crackers and mix with melted butter; sprinkle on top. Bake at 350 degrees for 30 minutes.

Shrimp Enchiladas

2 sticks butter
1 cup minced onion
1 cup canned green chilies, chopped
¾ cup bell pepper, minced
2¾ tsp. salt
2¾ tsp. white pepper
1½ tsp. cayenne
¾ tsp. dried oregano
½ tsp. garlic, minced

3 cups heavy cream
1 cup sour cream
8 cups shredded Monterey Jack cheese
2 pounds large cooked shrimp,
   cleaned and peeled
⅔ cup chopped green onions
½ cup cooking oil
20 corn tortillas, 6-inch

Melt one stick butter in skillet and sauté onion, chilies, and bell pepper. Mix in 1¼ tsp. salt, ¾ tsp. white pepper, ½ tsp. cayenne, ¼ tsp. oregano and ¼ tsp. garlic. Cook 10 minutes, stirring often. Stir in cream and bring to a rapid boil; reduce heat and simmer, stirring constantly for 10 minutes. Add sour cream and whisk about 3 minutes to mix well. Add 3 cups cheese and stir to melt. Set sauce aside.

Melt remaining 1 stick butter in 4-quart saucepan. Add cleaned shrimp, green onions, and remaining seasonings. Sauté about 6 minutes. Add cheese sauce. Heat through and set aside. Using small skillet and tongs, dip each tortilla into hot oil—just long enough to soften—and drain on paper towels. Put ⅓ cup sauce in each tortilla, roll up, and place (seam side down) on oven-safe serving platter. Cover with additional sauce and sprinkle with cheese. Melt cheese under broiler in 350 degree oven for about 5 minutes.

Tip: This sauce is great over spaghetti, rice, or noodles too!

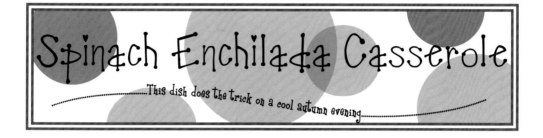

Spinach Enchilada Casserole

.......This dish does the trick on a cool autumn evening.......

2 lb. ground chuck
1 cup finely chopped onion
1 (16 oz.) can chopped tomatoes, very well drained
1 (12 oz.) pkg. frozen spinach, thawed, very well drained and dried
salt and pepper to taste
1 (10.75 oz.) can cream of mushroom soup
1 (10.75 oz.) can golden mushroom soup

1 (8 oz.) container sour cream
¼ cup milk
¼ tsp. garlic powder
1 stick butter, melted
16 corn tortillas
2 (4 oz.) cans chopped green chilies
2½ cups shredded cheddar cheese, divided
1 small can sliced black olives, very well drained

In a large saucepan, cook meat until it loses its color, then drain. Crumble into large bowl and stir in onion, tomatoes, spinach, salt, and pepper; set aside. Be sure that all vegetables are as well drained as possible to avoid watering down the flavors.

In another bowl, mix soups, sour cream, milk, and garlic powder together and set aside.

Gently melt butter in a 10-inch skillet. Dip half the tortillas in melted butter. Arrange on bottom and up sides of 9×13 inch baking dish. Spoon in half of meat mixture. Spread 1 can of chilies and 1 cup of the cheese over meat. Dip remaining tortillas in melted butter and make a second layer. Drop the sour cream sauce over the top, smoothing over entire surface. Cover with plastic wrap; refrigerate overnight.

Remove from refrigerator. Sprinkle with remaining ½ cup of cheese and sliced olives. Bake at 325 degrees for 35–40 minutes. Serve with whole black olives, salsa, and pickled jalapeño slices on the side.

Stuffed Pork Chops

1 stick butter
1 (6 oz.) pkg. of bread stuffing (like Mrs. Cubbison's)
1 (8 oz.) pkg. sliced crimini mushrooms
1 onion, diced
2 tender stalks celery, diced
½ small bell pepper, diced
½ tsp. salt
½ tsp. pepper
6 pork chops, 1 inch thick

Melt butter in large, deep skillet. Add stuffing, mushrooms, onion, celery, bell pepper, salt, and pepper; cook over low heat until bread is toasted and vegetables are wilted. Slice pocket into side of pork chops and season well (inside and out) with your favorite spices. Stuff with dressing and fasten with toothpicks.

Bake in uncovered casserole for 1 hour at 350 degrees.

Swiss Chicken Bliss

Chicken

  5 skinless, boneless chicken breasts,
     halved
  salt
  2 beaten eggs
  1 cup fine dry bread crumbs
  ½ stick butter

Sauce

  ½ stick butter
  ¼ cup flour
  ½ tsp. salt
  ⅛ tsp. pepper
  2½ cups milk
  ½ cup apple or white grape juice
  1 cup shredded Swiss cheese, more
     if desired
     avocado slices and tomato wedges
     for garnish

Place each chicken half between two pieces of wax paper and pound out to about ¼ inch thickness. Sprinkle lightly with salt. Dip each chicken piece into beaten eggs, then into crumbs. In skillet, heat 2 Tbsp. butter and brown a few chicken cutlets at a time (about 2 minutes on each side). Add remaining butter as needed until all 10 cutlets are browned. Set aside.

In saucepan, melt butter; blend in flour, salt, and pepper. Add milk all at once; cook and stir until thick and bubbly. Remove from heat; stir in juice. Pour about half the sauce into a 13×9×2 baking dish. Arrange chicken cutlets on top of sauce. Top with remaining sauce.

Bake covered in 350-degree oven about 50 minutes. Sprinkle with cheese. Top with avocado and tomato and return to oven for 3–5 minutes or until cheese is melted.

Yield: 8–10 servings.

Tuna Bake

1 stick butter
1 (8 oz.) pkg. white mushrooms, sliced
1 red pepper, diced
½ cup green pepper, diced
½ cup white wine or white grape juice
1 clove garlic, crushed
1 tsp. dry mustard
½ cup flour
   salt and pepper to taste
1 pint milk
2 (6.5 oz.) cans of albacore tuna, chunked
1 (14 oz.) pkg. macaroni shells, cooked and rinsed
1 (16 oz.) pkg. shredded sharp cheddar cheese

Melt butter in large, deep skillet; sauté mushrooms and diced peppers until slightly tender; stir in white wine (or white grape juice) and garlic. Simmer for just a few minutes until wine (or juice) has mostly evaporated. Stir in dry mustard, flour, salt, and pepper to create a roux. Whisk in milk and heat until thickened. Add tuna and pasta.

Transfer to a large casserole dish; cover with cheese and bake at 350 degrees for 30–40 minutes until bubbly.

Wednesday Night Stroganoff

This dish is quick, but good enough to serve that "surprise" special guest for dinner

2 lb. tenderloin steak
1 stick butter
2 medium onions, thinly sliced
1 lb. fresh mushrooms, sliced
4 Tbsp. dry sherry or beef stock
  salt and pepper to taste
1 pint sour cream

Trim fat from steak and cut into thin strips about 2×½ inches. Set aside.

Place ½ stick butter in large skillet over medium-low heat; add onion. Cook gently for a few minutes until onion is softened. Add mushrooms and cook for 2–3 minutes more, stirring occasionally. Remove onions and mushrooms from pan and set aside.

Melt remaining butter in skillet and add steak strips. Cook gently, stirring frequently so that the meat cooks through (5–10 minutes). Return onion and mushrooms to pan. Add sherry or beef stock; season with salt and pepper to taste. Lower heat, stir in sour cream and mix gently until heated through. Serve immediately over white rice or buttered noodles.

Yield: 8 hearty servings.

Sides

CREAMY COTTAGE CHEESE DELIGHT
CREAMY HOMESTYLE MACARONI & CHEESE
FETTUCCINE ALFREDO
HEARTLAND FRIED RICE
MUSHROOM PILAF
SPAGHETTI BASILICO
APPLE STUFFING

"Fish, to taste good, must swim three times: in water, in butter, and in wine."....................Cooking proverb

Creamy Cottage Cheese Delight

1 lb. mozzarella cheese, shredded
1 cup flour
1 cup milk
1 (16 oz.) container cottage cheese
6 eggs, lightly beaten
1 tsp. Italian seasoning
1 stick butter, melted
1 tomato, thinly sliced

Combine mozzarella cheese, flour, milk, cottage cheese, eggs, and *half* of melted butter. Spread remaining half of melted butter in a 11×7 inch baking dish. Pour mixture into dish and decorate top with single layer of tomato slices.

Place cookie sheet under dish to guard against spills and bake at 375 degrees for 50 minutes to 1 hour. Let sit for 10 minutes to firm.

Yield: 12–15 servings.

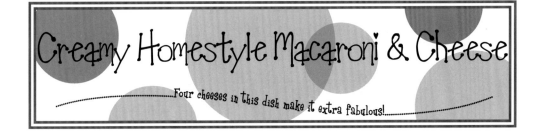

Creamy Homestyle Macaroni & Cheese

Four cheeses in this dish make it extra fabulous!

Macaroni
- 6 quarts water
- 1 lb. elbow macaroni
- ½ stick butter, divided
- 1 clove garlic, minced
- 3 Tbsp. flour
- ¼ tsp. Tabasco sauce, more if desired
- 3 cups milk
- ½ cup heavy cream

- 2 cups shredded sharp cheddar cheese
- 1 cup shredded Pepper Jack cheese
- 1 cup shredded Mozzerella cheese
- 1 tsp. salt
- ½ tsp. freshly ground pepper
- ½ tsp. dry mustard

Topping
- ½ stick butter
- 2½ cups dry bread crumbs
- ¾ cup Parmesan cheese
- 2 Tbsp. chopped fresh parsley

Preheat oven to 375 degrees.

Grease a 13×9 inch casserole dish. Cook the macaroni al dente; drain and stir in 1 Tbsp. butter. Set aside.

In a large saucepan, melt the remaining 3 Tbsp. butter. Add garlic and sauté for 1 minute. Add flour, and whisk until it begins to bubble. Add Tabasco and gradually whisk in milk; bring sauce to a boil. Reduce the heat to low and gradually add the cream, cheeses, salt, pepper, and mustard, whisking until the cheese melts and sauce is smooth. Taste the sauce for seasoning and add additional salt, pepper, or Tabasco if necessary. Stir the sauce into the macaroni, and transfer the mixture to prepared baking dish.

To make topping, melt butter in small pan on stovetop. Add bread crumbs and toss until well buttered, then add cheese and parsley, stirring to combine. Spread topping over casserole. Bake 30 minutes or until topping is golden.

Fettuccine Alfredo

Serve with grilled steak or chicken and fresh cut green beans—delicious!

1 (12 oz.) box fettuccine noodles
1 stick butter
3 cloves garlic, chopped
1 cup heavy cream, at room temperature
1 egg, at room temperature
¾ cup shredded Romano cheese
¼ cup chopped fresh parsley
   salt and pepper to taste

Cook fettuccine according to package directions. Drain well and place in a large, warm serving dish. Melt butter in medium large saucepan and sauté garlic. In separate bowl, mix egg with cream; add shredded cheese then slowly add to butter and garlic. Stir constantly until well combined; add parsley and seasonings. Pour over fettuccine and toss to coat. Serve immediately.

Heartland Fried Rice

One of the nice things about this dish is that you can go crazy with add-ins............
....I've provided a quick list to help get you going!

Fried Rice
- 5 eggs
- 1 stick butter
- 3 cups cooked white rice, unsalted and cooled
- ¼ cup finely minced fresh onion
- ¼ cup finely diced celery
- ¼ cup soy sauce

Add-ins
- cubed chicken
- frozen peas
- sugar snap peas
- cubed carrots
- mushrooms
- green onions

Melt 2 Tbsp. butter in large skillet. Add the fresh onion and celery, cook until just soft. Break eggs into a bowl and whisk together. Pour eggs into skillet with onion and celery and scramble until firmly set, breaking the eggs up into small pieces.

Add remaining butter, soy sauce, and rice. Cook over medium high heat for about 20 minutes, turning rice over occasionally.

Yield: 6 servings.

Tip: Add-ins should be cut into small and uniform pieces for even cooking. Toss them in at the same time as the onions and celery . . . and don't forget to check your leftovers for add-in possibilities!

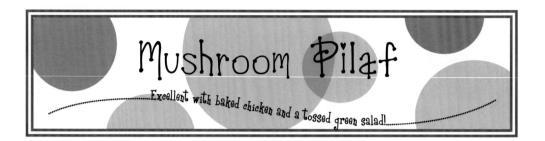

Mushroom Pilaf

Excellent with baked chicken and a tossed green salad!

    1 stick butter
    1 cup bulgur wheat
    1 cup vermicelli, broken into small pieces
4–5 large fresh mushrooms, sliced
    2 cups chicken stock (canned or homemade)
    1 bunch green onions, chopped fine

Over medium heat, melt butter in a large frying pan. Add the bulgur wheat, vermicelli, and sliced mushrooms; cook until vermicelli is slightly browned.

While the mixture in skillet is browning; bring the chicken broth to a boil. Carefully pour the broth over browned bulgur mixture. Add chopped green onions.

Remove from heat and spoon into large casserole dish with cover. Bake in covered casserole dish 30–35 minutes at 350 degrees. Remove cover after about 15 minutes.

Yield: 6–8 servings.

Spaghetti Basilico

A versatile side dish that makes a delicious complement for steak, barbecued chicken, or sautéed shrimp.

1 (1 lb.) pkg. spaghetti noodles
1 stick butter
1 large clove garlic, crushed
2 Tbsp. dried sweet basil
1 Tbsp. dried parsley flakes
½ tsp. salt
   pepper to taste
   shredded fresh Parmesan cheese to taste

Boil pasta in salted water until done per package instructions. While pasta is cooking, make sauce.

In large pan, melt butter over medium heat, add garlic and cook until transparent (1–2 minutes). Stir in basil and parsley; remove from heat.

Drain pasta and add salt, pepper, and Parmesan cheese; blend in seasoned butter mixture, stirring well.

Yield: 4–6 servings.

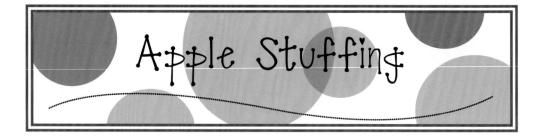

Apple Stuffing

    7 cups bread cubes
    3 cups diced Granny Smith apples
    1 cup minced onion
    1 cup seedless raisins
 1½ tsp. salt
 1¼ cups sugar
   ¼ tsp. pepper
    1 stick butter, melted
      turkey or chicken broth to moisten if needed

In a large bowl, stir all ingredients (except butter) together, being careful not to break up bread cubes. Pour butter over stuffing mixture and blend lightly.

If you'd like a little more moisture, use a few tablespoons of broth. Place stuffing into a lightly greased 2½- to 3-quart casserole dish. Cover and bake for 30–40 minutes at 325 degrees. If you'd like the top to be crunchy, uncover and bake for an additional 10–15 minutes.

Snacks

Crunchy Autumn Jumble
Heritage Honey Grahams
Nana's Caramel Corn
Sugared Fairy Pecans

Fancy hotel butter is 2 Tbsp. butter and 1 tsp. chopped parsley, ⅛ tsp. pepper, and 1 tsp. lemon juice; knead together and serve spread on steak or fish.—Revised from *Let's Cook*

Crunchy Autumn Jumble

  1 cup butter flavored syrup (like Mrs. Butterworth's)
½ cup sugar
  1 stick butter
½ tsp. cinnamon
10 cups crispy cereal (like Chex or Crispix)
  2 cups walnut halves
  2 cups pecan halves

Put syrup, sugar, butter, and cinnamon in a saucepan and bring to a boil over medium high heat, stirring often. Lower heat and simmer 2 minutes without stirring.

Mix cereal and nuts together in large bowl. Carefully pour sauce over dry ingredients and mix with large spoons or tongs.

Spray 2 cookie sheets lightly with oil. Spread mixture on the cookie sheets and bake at 250 degrees for 1 hour. Stir every 15 minutes.

Store in airtight containers or ziplock bags.

Tip: I find that mixing the cereal in last helps preserve the shape. Since cereals crumble easily, just use extra loving care when blending it in with everything else—otherwise you'll have lots of crumbs!

Heritage Honey Grahams

Who says you can't make these at home? Delicious when used as the cookies for ice cream sandwiches.

    1 stick very soft butter
    2 unbeaten eggs
    ½ cup honey
    2 tsp. vanilla
    ½ tsp. salt
  2¼ cups whole wheat flour

In a large bowl, mix together butter, eggs, honey, vanilla, and salt with large spoon. Leave butter in tiny pieces. Add the flour, a little at a time, until fully blended; let rest for 5 minutes.

Butter a large cookie sheet or jelly roll pan; place dough on sheet and pat it out until it's "graham cracker thin." Cover with wax paper and finish smoothing out with a rolling pin or glass tumbler. Smooth it out as close to the edges as possible. Remove paper; score into cracker-size squares. Prick each cracker with a fork several times just like those you get out of the package. Bake at 350 degrees for 15–20 minutes.

Nana's Caramel Corn

6 quarts popped popcorn (do not use microwave popcorn)
¼ tsp. cream of tartar
1 tsp. salt
1 tsp. baking soda
2 sticks butter
½ cup white corn syrup
2 cups brown sugar

Measure cream of tartar, salt, and baking soda into a small dish; set aside.

Combine butter, corn syrup, and brown sugar in a large saucepan. Bring to boil over medium high heat. Continue to slowly boil for 6 minutes, stirring constantly. Remove from heat.

Add cream of tartar, salt, and soda to caramel sauce and stir until well blended. Put popped popcorn into a very large bowl and very carefully pour hot caramel mixture over all. Mix well and spread out onto a buttered cookie sheet or two. Bake 1 hour at 200 degrees, stirring once after 30 minutes.

Serve warm or cool with apple juice or warm apple cider. Store in Ziplock bags.

Tip: Recipe may be easily cut in half.

Sugared Fairy Pecans

...Use these over salads, as snacks, or sprinkled on an ice cream sundae!...

     1 stick butter
     2 egg whites
     1 cup brown sugar
        salt
     1 tsp. cinnamon
  1½ lb. pecan halves

Melt butter in 9×13 pan in a 350 degree oven. Beat egg whites until stiff; add brown sugar, pinch of salt, cinnamon, and pecans. Bake ½ hour, stirring every 8–10 minutes. Cool and break apart.

Soups & Sauces

"Sea-Plain" Chowder
Heart-Warming Garlic & Potato Soup
Shrimp & Almond Cream Sauce
Meat & Cheese Mustard Sauce

When making butter balls, keep melon-baller in hot water and immediately drop shaped ball into cold water. Store in water in refrigerator until needed.

"Sea-Plain" Chowder

Filled with clams from the American coastline and corn from the Great Plains, this soup has an impressive flavor. The credit goes to my creative sister for having the imagination to name this one!

½ cup chopped onion
1 stick butter
4 Tbsp. flour
1 tsp. curry powder
8 cups fresh or frozen corn (uncooked)
8 cups milk
2 cups cream
   salt and pepper to taste
2 lbs. clam meat (preferably lump)

In a large pot (very large if you're making the whole recipe!), sauté onion in butter over medium heat until soft. Stir in flour and curry powder and cook 1 minute, stirring constantly. Add corn and cook 5 more minutes, stirring often. Slowly add milk, cream, salt, and pepper. Bring to boil over medium to medium-high heat. Continue to stir frequently.

Stir in clam meat and serve at once from the pot with toasted garlic bread. Top with shredded cheddar cheese and chopped parsley if desired.

Yield: 20 servings, but easily can be halved.

Heart-Warming Garlic & Potato Soup

8 medium potatoes, peeled and cubed
2 stalks celery, diced
1 medium onion, chopped
4 cups chicken broth
1 stick butter
3 cloves garlic, chopped
¼ cup flour
2 tsp. salt
½ tsp. pepper
4 cups milk

In soup kettle, combine potatoes, celery, onion, water, and chicken broth; bring to a boil. Reduce heat; cover and simmer 20 minutes or until potatoes are tender. Cool slightly. Place half of potato mixture in blender and puree. Blend remaining half to preferred consistency; set aside.

In the same kettle, melt butter and add chopped garlic. Stir in flour, salt, and pepper until smooth. Gradually add milk; bring to boil. Boil for 2 minutes. Return potato mixture to kettle and heat through.

Tip: Garnish with dollops of sour cream, crispy crumbled bacon, sharp cheddar cheese, and chopped parsley.

Shrimp & Almond Cream Sauce

Goes great over biscuits, buttered noodles, or rice!

    2 lbs. peeled and deveined shrimp
    1 stick butter
    ¼ cup brandy
    3 cups half and half
    ½ tsp. paprika
    3 cloves garlic, crushed
       salt and pepper to taste
    1 cup browned whole almonds
    ¼ cup chopped chives

In large, deep skillet, sauté shrimp in melted butter until shrimp begins to turn pink. Add brandy and light with match. When the alcohol burns off, add half and half. Simmer, stirring often, until thick. Season with paprika, garlic, salt, and pepper. Add almonds and sprinkle with chives before serving. Keep hot over hot water. Serve over biscuits, buttered noodles, or rice.

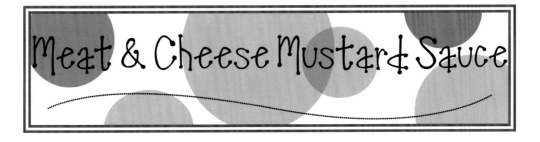

Meat & Cheese Mustard Sauce

4 oz. dry mustard
1 cup white vinegar
6 eggs, beaten separately
¾ cup light brown sugar
1 stick butter
½ small can of chopped jalapeño peppers

Mix mustard into vinegar and let sit for several hours. Pour into top of double boiler over hot water and whisk in eggs one at a time. Add brown sugar and butter. Cook over low heat for 7 minutes or until thick. Do not overcook or eggs will separate. Add jalapeño peppers last. Serve with meat or cheese cubes.

Yield: 1 quart.

Vegetables

Crispy Oven-Baked Potato Wedges
Fresh Herb & Garlic Potatoes
Mayberry Corn Bake
Potato Sour Cream Supreme
Sweet Corn Fritters with Herbed Sour Cream

To serve herbed butter, cut into pats, mold into shapes, or use a melon-baller to create butter spheres you can easily roll in dried herbs, spices, or finely chopped nuts.

Crispy Oven-baked Potato Wedges

These are tasty served with sour cream and chopped chives.

6–8 russet potatoes, scrubbed
1 stick butter
2 tsp. salt
½ cup dried bread crumbs
1 tsp. sugar

Parboil unpeeled potatoes until medium tender; drain. Cool slightly; peel and quarter lengthwise.

Melt butter in glass pie pan in microwave; add salt, bread crumbs, and sugar. Roll halved potatoes, a few at a time, into crumb mixture, coating well. Put into a 7×11 inch pan. Bake 15–20 minutes in 375 degree oven or until crispy.

Tip: Adding ¼ cup shredded Parmesan cheese to the coating mixture and using herbed bread crumbs makes these wedges perfect to serve with marinated meats—like Rosemary-infused ribeyes!

Fresh Herb & Garlic Potatoes

...The smaller the new potatoes the better...

16 small new potatoes
1 stick butter, cut in half
¼ cup olive oil
1 garlic clove, crushed and chopped
½ cup fresh chopped parsley
1 tsp. salt
½ tsp. pepper

Parboil potatoes for 5 minutes; drain and cover.

Melt half the stick butter and ¼ cup olive oil together in large skillet over medium heat. Sauté potatoes until tender and golden, turning frequently. If needed, bring heat up to medium high in order to get a nice crispy skin.

While potatoes are browning, melt remaining half stick butter in small saucepan. Add garlic and sauté over low heat until garlic has softened but not browned (1–2 minutes). Remove from heat; cool slightly and add parsley, salt, and pepper. Set aside.

When potatoes are tender and crisp, remove from skillet with slotted spoon and place in serving bowl. Pour garlic/parsley butter over all and toss lightly.

Serve with your choice of toppings: sour cream, bacon bits, chopped ham, or minced fresh herbs.

Yield: 4 servings.

Tip: Fresh herbs like parsley can easily be chopped up with help from a small bowl and your kitchen shears. Just toss the herbs in the bowl and snip-snip-snip.

Mayberry Corn Bake

...This sounds like something Aunt Bee would have fixed for Opie....

1 (4.75 oz.) can corn, well drained
1 (4.75 oz.) can cream style corn
1 stick butter, melted
1 cup cubed Velveeta
1 cup small macaroni, cooked al dente
2 Tbsp. finely chopped onion
½ lb. or more bacon, fried and crumbled

In a large bowl, mix both cans of corn with butter, cheese, macaroni, and onions. Bake in covered casserole dish at 350 degrees for 30 minutes. Uncover and sprinkle on bacon; bake for another half hour. Add a dash of hot sauce if you like a little zip!

Tip: There's not a lot of liquid in this dish so it's important that you boil the macaroni so it gets just the slightest head start on the baking process.

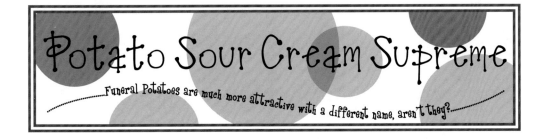

Potato Sour Cream Supreme

Funeral Potatoes are much more attractive with a different name, aren't they?

  1 (32 oz.) pkg. frozen hash browns, thawed
⅓–½ cup chopped green onions
  1 pt. sour cream
  1 can cream of chicken soup
  1 stick butter, melted
    salt and pepper to taste
  1 cup shredded cheese
  crushed potato chips or corn flakes

Mix ingredients in a large bowl. Bake in 9×13 pan at 350 degrees for 45 minutes to 1 hour until browned on top.

If you need a little more butter, then melt some and mix into crushed potato chips or corn flakes. Just use enough butter to moisten your chips or flakes and use to top this casserole with a crunchy finale.

Sweet Corn Fritters
with Herbed Sour Cream

2 (17 oz.) cans cream style corn
1 stick butter, melted
1 Tbsp. flour
3 Tbsp. sugar
½ tsp. salt
4 eggs, beaten
1 cup milk

Mix all ingredients together. Bake in lightly greased 1½-quart casserole dish at 350 degrees for 50 minutes. Serve with a dollop of herbed sour cream.

Herbed sour cream is as simple as finely chopping your favorites from the garden. I like parsley and basil mixed into my full fat sour cream. The full fat version tends to be firmer and make a prettier presentation.

Sources

Abrams, H. Leon. *Vegetariunism: An Anthropological/Nutritional Evaluation*. Reprinted in *Nourishing Traditions: The cookbook that challenges politically correct nutrition and the diet dictocrats*, revised 2nd ed., by Sally Fallon. Winona Lake, IN: New Trends Publishing, 2000.

Arkin, Frieda. *Kitchen Wisdom*. New York: Holt, Rinehart and Winston, 1977.

Douglass, William Campbell, MD. *The Milk Book*. Reprinted in *Nourishing Traditions*.

Fallon, Sally. *Nourishing Traditions: The cookbook that challenges politically correct nutrition and the diet dictocrats*, revised 2nd ed. Winona Lake, IN: New Trends Publishing, 2000.

Hawkins, Nancy. *Let's Cook*. New York: Alfred A. Knopf, 1943.

Lancet. 1994 344:1195.

PPNF Health Journal. Reprinted in *Nourishing Traditions*.

Price, Weston, DDS. *Nutrition and Physical Degeneration*. Reprinted in *Nourishing Traditions*.

Rubin, Hank. *The Kitchen Answer Book*. Capital Books, 2002.

Valentine, Tom. *Facts on Fats and Oils*. Reprinted in *Nourishing Traditions*.

Recipe Index

Recipe Index

About the Author

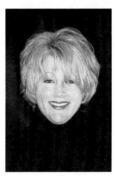

Angel collects cookbooks—thousands of them. Her favorites are the down-home community fundraising cookbooks with heritage recipes passed on joyfully for generations. One of the most common ingredients in all of these cookbooks is butter—wholesome, farm-fresh, flavorful butter.

With all the negative press that butter gets these days, it's no wonder that her fondness for nostalgia brought her to the conclusion that butter didn't have to be "badder"—it could be better! Friends, family, and co-workers urged her to bring her passion for butter to everyone by putting together a butter cookbook with love. You have in your hand the result.

After almost 30 years' worth of radio and television experience, Angel's weekly schedule includes cooking on ABC4's Good Things Utah or whipping up a dish on the radio at 94.1 KODJ. Her recipes have been printed in the Salt Lake Tribune newspaper and seen by 240,000 readers every week, and Angel's personal recipe website received over 167,000 hits in one month. She's active in cooking demonstrations at local home shows, markets, festivals, and fairs.

Angel lives in Salt Lake City with her husband Dickie and their cat Scooter (who's also a butter-lover).